The Virtues in Medical Practice

THE VIRTUES IN
MEDICAL PRACTICE

Edmund D. Pellegrino, M.D.
David C. Thomasma, Ph.D.

New York   Oxford
OXFORD UNIVERSITY PRESS
1993

Oxford University Press

Oxford   New York   Toronto
Delhi   Bombay   Calcutta   Madras   Karachi
Kuala Lumpur   Singapore   Hong Kong   Tokyo
Nairobi   Dar es Salaam   Cape Town
Melbourne   Auckland   Madrid

and associated companies in
Berlin   Ibadan

Published by Oxford University Press, Inc.,
200 Madison Avenue, New York, New York 10016

Oxford is a registered trademark of Oxford University Press

Library of Congress Cataloging-in-Publication Data
Pellegrino, Edmund D., 1920–
The virtues in medical practice /
by Edmund D. Pellegrino and David C. Thomasma.
p. cm.   Includes bibliographical references and index.
ISBN 0-19-508289-3
1. Medical ethics.   I. Thomasma, David C., 1939–   .   II. Title.
[DNLM: 1. Bioethics.   2. Ethics, Medical.   3. Philosophy, Medical.
W 50 P386v]
R724.P34   1993
174′.2—dc20
DNLM/DLC for Library of Congress   92-49073

3 5 7 9 8 6 4 2

Printed in the United States of America
on acid-free paper

We dedicate this book to our wives,
Clementine Pellegrino and Doris Thomasma,
as well as to our children:
Thomas, Stephen, Virginia, Michael, Andrea, Alice,
and Leah Pellegrino, Pieter and Lisa Thomasma,
and Emily and Stephanie Kulpa.

Acknowledgments

We wish to thank Marti Patchell and Doris Thomasma for their help in making the arrangements that brought about this book, as well as the help of David Miller in finding references, checking the text, and typing the initial text into the computer. Each of them provided us with irreplaceable patience, good humor, and meticulousness in dealing with our endless drafts and redrafts. All three persons are invaluable in supporting everything we do. We are very grateful to them. Also we thank the Rev. Joseph Daniel Cassidy, O.P., for his meticulous help in proofreading the manuscript.

One of us (E. D. Pellegrino) wishes to express gratitude to the Rockefeller Foundation which provided support for a period as resident scholar at the Villa Serbelloni in Bellagio, Italy, during September 1988. A significant part of this book was completed there. No more congenial setting or support for a scholarly endeavor can be imagined. The other of us (D. C. Thomasma) wishes to thank Loyola University of Chicago for its support through a leave of absence from July 1991 through December of that year, which permitted him to complete initial drafts of portions of the book.

Contents

Human society owes its strength and vitality
to the intrinsic virtue of its members.

George Santayana, *Dominations and Powers*, p. 3.

Introduction

Until very recently, ethics in general and biomedical ethics in particular have been largely principle-based. Virtue-based ethics was given scant attention. Yet for most of its history, the emphasis of ethics was on living a good life and becoming a good person, that is to say, on the acquisition of certain desirable characteristics we call the virtues. Indeed, the ancient codes of medical ethics—Greek, Indian, and Chinese—were virtue-based. Their prescriptions and proscriptions looked to the character of the physician as the final guarantee of the well-being of the patient and as the basis of professional standards and practices. The same can be said of the ethics of Thomas Percival and his eighteenth-century colleagues, James and John Gregory, who so heavily influenced the first ethical code of the American Medical Association.[1]

Elizabeth Anscombe and Alasdair MacIntyre, followed by many other contemporary ethicists, have recently been reexamining virtue ethics, remining and redefining the riches of this tradition in philosophy.[2,3] The result has been a veritable renaissance of interest in virtue, the virtues, and the virtuous person. A similar refurbishment of virtue in the writings of bioethicists has just begun.[4] It promises to be as significant as the effort in general ethics.

In part, the interest stems from a desire to enrich principle-based ethics, which has enjoyed such success. Recently principle-based ethics has come under fire for its almost formulaic approach to ethics. Based, as it is, on the application of the principles of autonomy, beneficence, and justice to individual cases, this form of ethics fails to take into sufficient account the character of the agent, as well as the nuances of real life that situate and define the moral quandary. While incomplete, a principle-based ethic nonetheless has much to offer, not the least of which is its freedom from the slavery of the moment in favor of a more universalizable view. Standards and guidelines against which individuals, institutions, and society can measure their actions are necessary. But they must be linked to a virtue-based ethic if a more complete picture of the moral life is to be obtained.

Fortunately, there is a new openness to the ethics of virtue in today's ethical discourse. This openness stems in part from the successes of principle-based ethics and in part from some of its deficiencies. In part, too, it stems from the growing experience of ethicists in the clinical setting. In that setting it is obvious that the way principles are selected, interpreted, ordered in relation to each other, and applied, is dependent on the character of each participant in a clinical activity.

Efforts to combine a virtue ethic with principled ethical theories are laudable but have so far been less than successful. Beauchamp and Childress have made a serious attempt, but in the end they largely concentrate on the principles.[5] They do point out that virtue theory has a special place in moral deliberation in health care, but argue that it cannot replace duty-based ethics:

> The special role of virtues in ethical theory should not be construed as evidence for a primary role, as if a virtue-based theory were more important than or could replace obligation-based theories. The two kinds of theory have different emphases, but they are compatible and mutually reinforcing.[6]

James Drane and William Ellos make a stronger case than this for the place of virtues in medical ethics, as we shall see later.[7]

Our approach differs from those we have mentioned in one important respect. The other efforts link virtue theory with principle-based theories without moving through the virtue of prudence, that is, establishing right reason in action, *recta ratio agibilium,* as St. Thomas called it.[8] More important, other theories neglect the intrinsic relationship between prudence, the other virtues, and the nature of medicine and professional dedication. Thus, virtue and principle-based theories in medical ethics must be closely linked with the nature of medicine itself, that is, with a philosophy of medicine. Our own previous efforts to construct a modern philosophy of medicine have led us to this conclusion and now have prompted us to write this book.[9]

Thus, this book represents an attempt to apply virtue theory to biomedical, particularly health professional, ethics. In this volume we explore the natural virtues, that is, the philosophical foundations of virtue-based ethics, their historical roots in the classical and medieval traditions, and the application of such theory to the practice of medicine today. Our approach here is teleological, in the Aristotelian and Thomistic sense, relating the virtues of medicine as a practice to the ends of medicine.

A philosophy of medicine is essential to any such virtue theory since it defines the ends toward which the virtues are directed and from which they derive their justification. Indeed, the choices of the virtues we examine and apply to medicine are made in the context of a philosophy of medicine. We have argued that the moral essence of a health profession is the special relationship that sickness and the response to illness creates between healer and patient.

For that reason, the virtues that interest us in this book are those that arise from the caring bond (which includes healing, caring, and curing) and the public trust implied by the commitment to care for another—faith and healing, trust, hope, compassion, courage, fidelity, and the like. There are many other virtues, of course. Our examination does not take all of them into account. Rather, the ones selected arise from the focus of our philosophy of medicine on the relation of doctor and patient. In effect we are paralleling the relation between ethical theory and applied ethics by selectively applying certain virtues to medical practice without necessarily accepting the theory that may originally have accompanied discussion of that virtue. Yet we are also interested in theoretical issues underlying the concept and practice of the virtues. From time to time at appropriate points, we will briefly look at such issues as well. In Chapter 2 we tackle the thorny problem of the relationship of the virtues to ethical principles and duties in medicine. In Chapter 13, we apply virtue ethics in medicine to see how they make a difference in the way current disputes are analyzed. Throughout we use case examples for the same purpose. And in Chapter 14, we focus on the problem of whether the medical virtues can be taught.

We wish to take into account a set of virtues entailed in being a good physician. We are thus positioned midway between theory and practice, as is the medical enterprise itself. For the most part we will adopt the realist, Thomist position in detailing the virtues but will use selective insights from other thinkers, as we have done in two previous works on the philosophy of medicine. This approach allows us to draw on the insights of various philosophers and moral theologians to illuminate further one or another feature of medical practice.

For those reasons, this book deals with the resurgence of interest in virtue ethics, specifically as it applies to medical ethics. It propounds the theses (1) that virtue is an irreducible element in medical ethics, (2) that virtue ethics must be redefined, however, to take into account the contributions of analytical, so-called quandary ethics, (3) that the virtues characteristic of the good physician are a fusion of general and special virtue ethics, (4) that, as in other professional and social roles, the virtues of medicine are derivable from the nature of medicine as a human activity, (5) that the derivation of the physician's virtues from the ends of medicine helps us to escape some of the difficulties inherent in a "free-standing" virtue ethic, (6) that some link must be made between principle-, duty-, and virtue-based ethics, and (7) that some link must be made between moral philosophy and moral psychology, that is, between cognition of the good and motivation to do the good.

These are philosophically ambitious projects with implications well beyond medical ethics. But our focus will be on medical ethics, on the healing relationship, the phenomenology of that relationship and the derivation of the characteristics of the good physicians from the nature of the kind of activity medicine is. The implications for questions outside medicine are left, for the most part, to the reader's interpretation. Suffice it to say that medicine provides a paradigm case for the exploration of virtue and character ethics and its relationship to the other theories that now dominate medical ethics.

After all the arguments are in place, we tend to accept the notion that there is a human nature, and that this nature, while developing physically and socially, transcends time and place sufficiently so that propositions can be made about it. Among the propositions are those embodied in medicine itself. Others are those that are developed over the centuries in ethics. Even if we grant that there are seemingly irreconcilable spheres or traditions of moral discourse, as MacIntyre would have it, there is sufficient linkage among human beings and human activity that individuals within each tradition can argue about the insights, assumptions, logic, and applicability of those in other systems of moral inquiry. While acknowledging the contribution of theological ethics both to medical ethics and to the debate about moral inquiry, this study confines itself to philosophical argumentation, refraining from recourse to scripture, religious tradition, or ecclesiastical authority.

This book is intended for physicians, philosophers interested in virtue theories, and the educated public concerned with the state of professional ethics. Practitioners in nursing and the other health professions will find much of what we discuss applicable by analogy to their own specialties. Clearly there are ethical issues specific to the other health professions that we have not explored. This is more properly done, in our opinion, by practitioners in those professions and ethicists working with them. We hope our exploration of the virtues in medical practice will stimulate them to a similar inquiry into nursing, social welfare, and the other health professions.

In these pages we urge refocusing medical ethics on the personhood of the physician and the patient, on the ancient search for the good human being. No matter what theory of ethics one espouses—principle, duty-based, casuistical, emotivist, situational, or intuitionist—the moral agent is a constant factor in the implementation of the moral act. Virtue, the virtues, and the virtuous person are unavoidable conceptions. These we hope to have clarified in this work.

Notes

1. Edmund D. Pellegrino, "Foreword: Thomas Percival, The Ethics Beneath the Etiquette," *Medical Ethics, or a Code of Institutions and Precepts Adapted to the Professional Conduct of Physicians and Surgeons, Thomas Percival, MD* [reprinted from the 1805 version] (Birmingham, AL: Classics of Medicine Library, 1985), pp. 1–65.

2. G. E. M. Anscombe, *Ethics, Religion, and Politics* (Minneapolis: University of Minnesota Press, 1981); *Plato, the Sophist and the Statesman* (New York: Thomas Nelson, 1961); and *From Parmenides to Wittgenstein* (Minneapolis: University of Minnesota Press, 1981).

3. Alasdair MacIntyre, *After Virtue,* 2d ed. (Notre Dame, IN: Notre Dame University Press, 1984).

4. James Drane, *Becoming a Good Doctor: The Place of Virtue and Character in Medical Ethics* (Kansas City, MO: Sheed and Ward, 1988).

5. Tom Beauchamp and James Childress, *Principles of Biomedical Ethics,* 3d ed. (New York: Oxford University Press, 1989), pp. 374–399.

6. Ibid., p. 379.

7. See 4; William Ellos, *Ethical Practice in Clinical Medicine* (London: Routledge, 1990).

8. For St. Thomas an act is moral if it is capable of being controlled by the will as agent. The possibility of freedom being ordered by truth must exist for an act to be moral, that is, ordering of reason is required to direct an act to good moral ends (*Summa Theologiae,* 1a 2ae, Q. 1–5). For Aquinas, the end determines the species of the moral act. This means that the end (sometimes the intention, sometimes the physical end of the action, sometimes the goal of the agent, sometimes all of the above) establishes the nature of the moral act itself, not necessarily the rectitude of the action, which is also subject to analysis in terms of other factors (objective evil of the act, extenuating circumstances, and the like). See Brian Thomas Mullady, O.P., *The Meaning of the Term "Moral" in St. Thomas Aquinas* (Vatican City: Libreria Editrice Vaticana, 1986).

9. See Edmund D. Pellegrino and David C. Thomasma, *A Philosophical Basis of Medical Practice* (New York: Oxford University Press, 1981); *For the Patient's Good: The Restoration of Beneficence in Health Care* (New York: Oxford University Press, 1988).

I

THEORY

1

Virtue Theory

Medicine is a moral community because it is at heart a moral enterprise and its members are bound together by a common moral purpose. If this is so, they must be guided by some shared source of morality—some fundamental rules, principles, or character traits that will define a moral life consistent with the ends, goals, and purposes of medicine. For centuries, this source was the character of the physician and, in keeping with the moral philosophy of the times, virtue ethics provided the conceptual foundation for professional ethics. In modern times, for reasons we shall outline briefly, virtue has been supplanted by principle- and rule-based ethics.

In this chapter, we shall examine the concept of virtue, its transformations in the post-medieval and modern periods, and its reemergence most recently in general and medical ethics. In the next chapter, we shall relate virtue-based and principle- or duty-based theories. Both chapters are part of a prolegomenon for the bulk of the book, which defines the virtues most specific to medicine, the way they delineate the character traits that the good physician should exhibit, and the way the virtues shape the practice of medicine.

The Concept of Virtue

The history of the concept of virtue may be conveniently divided into four periods: (1) the classical-medieval period, in which the virtues were central to all moral philosophies; (2) the post-medieval and modern periods, when virtue remained important but was reshaped by the emergence of new systems of moral philosophy; (3) the positivist-analytical period when virtue ethics was in decline, along with much of traditional normative ethics; and (4) the present period of resuscitation of virtue as a basis for morality. In each period, the concept of virtue was shaped by the dominant moral philosophy. Remnants of these philosophies may be found in the contemporary refurbishment of the concept of virtue. In general, however, the central notion of virtue and the virtues, even today, is rooted in the classical-medieval synthesis, particularly its roots in the *Nicomachean Ethics*, the *Eudemian Ethics*, and the *Magna Moralia* of Aristotle.

3

The Classical Period: Socrates, Plato, Aristotle

The definitions of virtue dominant in classical, medieval, and Renaissance moral philosophy had several ideas in common: they maintained that (1) the aim of philosophy was to teach how to live a good life; (2) virtue and the individual virtues were essential to being a good person and living a good life; (3) there were potentials in human nature, and virtue enabled human beings to fulfill them; (4) the virtues could be discovered by reason and were under the guidance of reason in their operation.

The concept of virtue originated in the Western world with the Greek philosophers. The Sophists prepared the way for the conceptions of Plato and Aristotle. They believed that virtue could be taught to any man and that they were essential for the exercise of power. For the Sophists, the virtues were a product of reason alone; what could not be explained by reason was not a virtue.[1]

It was Socrates who posed the fundamental questions about virtue with which moral philosophy has wrestled ever since. He has Meno say, "Can you tell me, Socrates, whether virtue is acquired by teaching or practice, or if by neither teaching nor practice, whether it comes to us by nature or some other way?" (*Meno* 70 a) Tantalizingly, Socrates did not answer these questions, and they haunt us today. Partial, and sometimes conflicting, answers appear in the other Platonic dialogues and in every subsequent attempt to clarify the notion of virtue.

Socrates did say, or Plato had him say, that virtue was knowledge, that is, knowledge of the good for humans. If men did not act well, it was because of ignorance. No one, he opined, would seek evil except through ignorance of the good. Wisdom (*Sophia*) thus became the virtue par excellence. Although he was skeptical of definitions of the individual moral virtues (*Laches* and *Charmides*), Plato recognized virtue itself as knowledge (*Episteme*) of the excellence (Arete) of the good life. The virtues themselves he saw as definable by the degree to which they conformed to the pure forms—justice, wisdom, and so on.

Characteristically, Plato in different dialogues examines contrary opinions. In the early dialogues he emphasized personal virtue, and in later dialogues the kind of society in which the good person could flourish. In the *Protagoras* and *Meno,* he argues against virtue as knowledge, for if virtue cannot be taught, it cannot be knowledge. In the *Euthydemus,* he takes the opposite viewpoint. In the *Republic,* the major emphasis is on justice. In his discussion of virtue Plato seemingly neglects feelings, passions, or emotions. The good is conceived as so attractive that vice can only mean that the good simply has not been recognized as such by the vicious man.

Plato's concern was to develop a general theory of virtue. While he did enumerate the "cardinal" virtues—fortitude, temperance, justice, and wisdom—he did not see ethics as a practical science in the way Aristotle did. Indeed, much of Aristotle's argumentation is a critique of Plato's attempt at generalization. Thus, in *The Politics* (1260 a 5), Aristotle warns of the deception in any general theory, and in the *Magna Moralia* (1182 a 20), he points out the omission in Socrates' theory of the place of the emotions. For Aristotle, the aim of ethics is practical—to be good and to act well (NE 1102 b 26; NE 1144 b 18).

Ethics thus seeks truth of a particular kind, truth about the ends of human actions—about happiness, which is the result of activity in accord with excellence (NE 1177 a 12 12–18). Ethics thus is the science of the pursuit of the individual goods, and politics of the social good. Individual good here does not mean selfish interest, but the good of the person *qua* person, of the person as a human being directed by nature to happiness. Happiness, in turn, is not synonymous with the pursuit of selfish interest—which may, indeed, be a vice.

Aristotle defines virtue as a "state of character" that "brings into good condition the thing of which it is the excellence and makes the work of that thing to be done well" (NE 1106 a 15–17). "Therefore, if this is true in every case, the excellence of human beings will also be a state of character which makes a person good and makes the person do his or her work well" (NE 1106 a 22–24). In equating virtue with character, Aristotle was being faithful to the Greek meaning of the word *ethiké*, which means "character."

Aristotle's whole inquiry into virtue is, as he says, "not in order to know what excellence is, but in order to become good. We must examine the nature of action, how we ought to do them. . . . The whole account of conduct, however, cannot be given precisely" (NE 1104 a). Aristotle proposes no rule book of morality but insists that "agents must in each case consider what is appropriate to the occasion as happens also in medicine or navigation" (NE 1104 a).

Aristotle's emphasis is on traits of character, not particular acts of an agent but the dispositions an agent habitually brings to his acts. Virtues are traits that make a person good and enable him to do his work well. They thus have a teleological quality in relation both to the person and to the "work" of living a good life.

Virtues also are concerned with choice. Recognition of the good does not ensure doing the good. Aristotle thus admits into consideration the passions or emotions in a way that Plato did not. The acts of the virtuous person proceed from three things: a knowledge of the good in any actions, a choice of the good for its own sake, and a source for knowledge and choice in a good character. It is the traits of good character that ensure that the right and good will not only be recognized but also chosen.

Virtue for Aristotle, therefore, is not just a feeling about what is good, or just a capacity to make a good choice. Virtue is a habitual disposition to act well. Virtue results from the habitual exercise of the virtues. Virtue thus can be taught by training and practice. Aristotle thereby answers one of Meno's questions to Socrates: virtues can be taught. While virtue has certain attributes of a habit, it is not a Pavlovian reflex. Virtue is a habit under the guidance of reason. It is not an automatic or unthinking reflex, or simply an intuitive response to innate knowledge of the good. It is here that the virtue of phronesis enters, a concept that we will discuss in more detail later.

Aristotle divides the virtues into the intellectual and the moral. The intellectual virtues are art, science, intuition, reasoning, and practical wisdom (*Nicomachean Ethics* 1139 b 16). They are related to the life of reason. There are other virtues appropriate to the moral life—the moral virtues. Most of the *Nicomachean Ethics* concerns itself with a detailed examination of specific moral virtues. Aristotle accepts the four cardinal virtues, as does Plato, but he adds others, like magnanimity.

The greatest weakness of Aristotle's theory of virtue is his doctrine of the mean. "Excellence is that state concerned with choice lying in a mean relative to us. This being determined in a way which the person of practical reason would determine it" (NE 1107 a 1). Obviously, not all virtues can be located as the mean between extremes. Can one be too just, for example?[2] Aristotle compounds the difficulty when he provides lists of the specific virtues, which vary in content in his other treatises. Aristotle agrees with Plato and Socrates on certain central virtues like justice, wisdom, and temperance. He lists others here and there, faltering when he moves from consideration of virtue in general to the virtues in particular. He is no more successful than Socrates in answering Meno's question of whether the virtues are one or many. He is consistent, however, with most other moral philosophers in defining the "core" or cardinal virtues. We do not think it necessary to defend the doctrine of the mean. Aristotle's theory of virtue can stand without it and can be the foundation upon which a contemporary ethic of virtue can be built—particularly as we wish to do in the ethics of medicine.

Aristotle's theory, which links moral decisions and the character of the agent, is very important to later moral theories that emphasize moral psychology. Linking virtues to character opens the way to connecting moral cognition, moral motivation, and moral action with each other. It also places the emphasis on the skills necessary to be a good person rather than the skills necessary to carry out professions or what von Wright calls "technical goodness."[3] In the chapters on the virtues in medical practice we will reexamine these connections more closely.

Aristotle goes well beyond Plato in centering ethics on virtue. Except for the weakness of his definition of virtue as a mean, Aristotle's conceptualization of virtue and its relationship to the good, to a philosophy of human nature, and to the emotions constitutes a coherent moral philosophy and a still viable conception of virtue and the virtuous person.

The Stoics

Equally influential with Aristotle and Plato in classical and medieval conceptions of virtue are the thinkers of the Early, Middle, and Late Stoa. During its 500-year history, Stoicism has exerted a major influence on the ethics of virtue. It shaped the ethics of the Hellenistic world and became the dominant moral philosophy of educated Romans. It influenced the early development of Christian ethics and inspired the idea of the educated gentleman of eighteenth-century England. The professional ethics of Stoic medical writers added elements of compassion and humanism to Hippocratic medical ethos.[4]

The ethics of the Stoa, like that of Aristotle, was linked to a theory of human nature and the good. The key to Stoic moral philosophy was its notion of nature and the laws of nature. Human beings are part of nature. They share in the divine creative force and in the necessity of accommodation to the laws of nature. The good and happiness of humanity reside in the benevolence and orderliness of nature, according to which man must live to be happy. This is the way to *apatheia* (absence of disturbing passions) and *euthymia* (spiritual peace and well-being).

The Stoics taught that the virtues are the means by which persons can reach these ends. By practicing the virtues, humanity can become free and benevolent, as God is free and benevolent. The key virtues are wisdom, courage, temperance, and justice—the same cardinal virtues taught by Plato and Aristotle. They are the attitudes that enable us to discern what is good and bad, what we should fear, how we should control our desires, and how to render to each his due. Benevolence has a particular place in Stoicism. All men are brothers under the fatherhood of God; even slaves are worthy of benevolence and justice. Indeed, a major obligation is to serve our fellows.[5]

Stoicism asserted that virtue was its own reward more forcefully than any other virtue-based ethical system. It also emphasized the notion of duty, particularly in the writings of the Roman Stoics like Seneca, Epictetus, and especially Cicero. Cicero's manual on duties, ''De Oficiis,'' exerted a strong influence on anyone with a classical education right up to modern times. In that work, Cicero transmitted the idea of role-specific duties, which Panaetius of Rhodes introduced during the period of the Middle Stoa. In the writings of the Stoics, it is difficult to separate the concept of duty from the concept of virtue. Adherence to duty seems almost to be the definition of virtue—very close to Kant's definition of virtue.

The Stoics also sought the wise man as a model of virtuous behavior. He was one who practiced the virtues, freed himself from wants, practiced serenity in the face of all hardships, and thus was free and independent of circumstances just like the Stoic God. Though the perfect wise man was a rarity, figures like Marcus Aurelius and Epictetus captured the imagination and inspired later generations even in our times.

This is not the place to trace the transformations of the classical conception of virtue, in either its Aristotelian or Stoic formulations in late antiquity. The history of the relationships of the older conception to the teachings of the later Platonists, Stoics, and thinkers in Judaism, Christianity, and Islam is complex. Each of these world views had its own definition of the nature of human life, its destiny, and the source of the principles that define the good life. These views interacted with and reshaped the classical idea. The notion of divine law and spiritual life became important determinants of what constitutes virtuous behavior. We wish to underline the roots of any virtue theory within the community that supports the individuals. Suffice it to say at this point that these interrelationships laid the groundwork for the next major exemplification of virtue ethic, which occurred in the Middle Ages— particularly in the ethics of Thomas Aquinas.

The Medieval Period

During the Middle Ages, the classical idea of virtue was refined by reconciling it with the virtue ethic of the Christian Gospels. The major figure in this synthesis was Thomas Aquinas. A large segment of his monumental *Summa Theologiae* is devoted to the ethics of virtue, which is central to his moral philosophy. This was consistent with his great enterprise of reconciling Aristotelian philosophy and Augustinian and scriptural theology.

Aquinas appropriated much of Aristotle's philosophy of the natural virtues and added to it the concept of the theological virtues, greatly expanded and enriched

Aristotle's conception of phronesis, and explored regions of moral psychology, like intentionality, that Aristotle merely hinted at.

For Aquinas, as for Aristotle, ethics was teleological. The moral quality of human acts derived from their relationship to the final end of human life. Virtues are habitual dispositions to perform actions that accord with this end. Like Aristotle, Aquinas gives reason an important place in virtue—"it belongs to human virtue to make a man good and his work according to reason" (S.T. 2–2ae, 122.1).

Since the ultimate end of human existence is spiritual, Aquinas taught that the natural virtues need to be completed by the supernatural virtues—faith, hope, and charity. These virtues are not, like the natural virtues, acquired by practice. They are directed to God as their end. Of the three supernatural virtues, charity is the ordering virtue. These two categories of virtues, the natural and the supernatural, are not in conflict since, in Aquinas' view, faith and reason complement each other.

Aquinas accepted the classical cardinal virtues as defined by Plato and Aristotle but gave special place to practical wisdom, or prudence. Prudence bridged the gap between the moral and intellectual virtues. It is the virtue that disposes the reason to fit the good end of an act. Virtue thus disposes one to integrate right intentions, right thinking, and right acting. Prudence has particular pertinence, as does intention in medical ethics, and we will take up these subjects later in this book.

Postmedieval Transformations

The concept of virtue underwent dramatic changes, and so did its place in moral philosophy as the Aristotelian-Thomist synthesis was repeatedly challenged in the philosophies of the postmedieval period. The story of these transformations is actually the story of the development of modern moral philosophy, and it is far too complex to be recounted here in any satisfactory way. It is useful, however, to sketch in some of the forces that reshaped the meaning of virtue in ways that exert powerful influence today.

The idea of virtue was so intimately enmeshed in Aristotelianism, Thomism, and Scholasticism that it suffered erosion as these systems of thought were challenged in the Renaissance and the Enlightenment. Some of the forces operating against the classical-medieval synthesis were the distrust of metaphysics and Scholastic methodologies and the limitations of Aristotelian science. Teleological and theological arguments lost ground as science and empiricism demonstrated what they could contribute to human knowledge by the experimental method.

Human nature distinguished by reason and definable in terms of some ultimate end gave way to more "realistic" approaches, the realistic anthropology of Hobbes' and Locke's recrafted ethics in terms of rights, the social contract, and individualism. Hume and his British colleagues moved the discussion of ethics into the realm of moral psychology as they explored the notion of an inherent moral sentiment that led humans to give approbation to some acts and not to others. Kant reconstructed the entire metaphysics of morals and recast the ancient Stoic notion of duty in terms of moral maxims and the categorical imperative. In contradiction of Hume and the British empiricists, he gave reason a central place in ethics. For Kant duty was performed because it was duty that defined the whole of morality, irrespective of the consequences. On the other hand, consequences were for Jeremy Bentham and John Stuart Mill the final determination of the moral quality of acts. Others, like the Cambridge Platonists, built their moral systems on intuitions of the good, and still others denied that the good was definable.

As one might suspect, with moral philosophy in such flux, the concepts of virtue were many, varied, and often contradictory. Almost every writer of importance had something to say about virtue, particularly during the period when study of the texts of the classical writers was revived. We will list a few examples to illustrate the confusing interpretations that followed the dissolution of the older conceptions of virtue.

Montaigne, for example, defined virtue as "an innocence accidental and fortuitous"; Descartes called it "strength of souls" and Malebranche "love of order." For Hume virtue was "a quality of mind agreeable to or approved by everyone who considers or contemplates it." Kant defined virtue as "a coincidence of the rational will with every duty firmly settled in the character." Duty was synonymous with respect for the categorical imperative, which Kant stated in two ways: "Act only according to that maxim whereby you can at the same time will that it should become a universal law" and "Act in such a way that you treat humanity, whether in your own person or in the person of another, always at the same time as an end and never simply as a means."[6] These injunctions apply irrespective of desires or consequences.

Kant's respect for person and Bentham and Mill's utility established the idea of a "principle-based" ethic as distinguished from the traditional emphasis on virtue. Ethics was set on the road of emphasis on the act more than on the agent even though, in Kant's case, intention was paramount in moral acts and therefore resided in the agent. Sidgwick's later refinement of utilitarianism made utility a self-evident principle apprehensible by common sense, without need of formal philosophical development. His work and that of Ross are the foundation for the dominant form of principle-based ethics today. This begins with a limited number of prima facie principles that are held to be normative unless good reason to the contrary can be adduced.

Antivirtue Theories

We shall have more to say about the move to principle-based ethics in the next chapter when we compare it with virtue-based ethics and suggest how principle and virtue might be linked. Now we need to complete our review of the transformations in the older concept of virtue that followed the sustained critique of both classical and medieval philosophy in the Renaissance and the Enlightenment. MacIntyre has summarized brilliantly the post-Enlightenment dissolution of the finely woven cloth of virtue-based ethics. Our aim is simply to mention the antivirtue strains in some philosophies and then to close this chapter with a sampling of some definitions of virtue emerging in our own day as the values of virtue-based ethics are becoming reappreciated.

The antivirtue strain appeared even as the classical definitions were being framed in Plato's dialogues. In the *Gorgias,* Callicles questions Socrates' insistence on the virtues as prerequisites for becoming a good person or forming a good society. Some see him as the forerunner of Nietzsche. Thrasymachus in the *Republic* poses another challenge to virtue, this time the virtue of justice. Justice, Thrasymachus argues, is determined by those in power. It has no other foundation or justification. In a similar vein, again in the *Republic*, Callicles and Glaucon both express skepticism about Socrates' theories of virtue in general and in particular—especially their importance for a good society.

Machiavelli's form of antivirtue thinking has a powerful appeal today because it asserts the difficulty of survival in a competitive society that lives by rules of nonvirtue. Macchiavelli advised his prince not to worry about the natural or the Christian virtues when it comes to the exercise of power. The security and well-being of the state were the prince's concern, and he should be cruel or magnanimous as the occasion demanded. No prince could make a profession of virtue and remain in power if the people and other princes were not virtuous. Instead, Macchiavelli espoused *virtu*—manliness, courage, military and political might—something closer to present-day machismo than to classical virtue.

Macchiavelli's cynicism about the survival value of virtue has a special appeal to many today, even in the professions that have traditionally made obeisance to virtue, like medicine, the law, and the ministry. Physicians and lawyers are increasingly of the opinion that virtue and ethics are fine ideals, but that they are impossible to follow in our competitive, free-market, bureaucratized society.

A particularly powerful brand of antivirtue ethics akin to Macchiavelli's and Hobbes' ethical pessimism is Ayn Rand's. Ms. Rand exalted the virtue of selfishness[7] and concluded, somewhat like Adam Smith, that if we could free the creative energies of self-interest, all would benefit. For Rand, honesty has value because it serves self-interest and survival, but it is not defensible in the way value theories would have it. A contemporary medical prototype of antivirtue ethics can be seen in the proposal by Engelhardt and Rie for a "new ethic" of medicine that would replace beneficence with self-interest. These authors argue that accommodation to the free-market approach to health care should be the basis for a needed revision of medical ethics. In fact, they suggest that skimming paying patients and dumping nonpaying patients on the public system of health care can be seen as a virtue, since this would force society to grapple with its own duties to the poor.[8] This view is so contrary to the views we are espousing that we shall not attempt a refutation here. It has not garnered the serious critique it deserves. Rather, at this point, if the argument of this book is in any way sound, it should provide its own rebuttal of this latest antivirtue theory of medical morals.

Before we leave the antivirtue construct, we must mention another physician antivirtue theorist, Bernard Mandeville. In his *Fable of the Bees,* Mandeville argues that vices like self-indulgence, love of luxury, and envy are really virtues. They make for profitable trade, employment, and productivity, thus ensuring that a society will thrive. When the bees in Mandeville's *Fable* turn to virtue, their hive no longer thrives. Similar strains of cynicism about virtue hover over other philosophies and in the public mind. They inevitably surface whenever virtue is espoused as a desirable goal for professional life or education.

The most powerful and sophisticated attack on the virtues as traditionally taught is that of Nietzsche. In his *Uebermensch,* he labels the virtues taught by Judaism and Christianity as the virtues of slaves and emasculated weaklings. Christian virtues for Nietzsche are therefore vices. They are of no account to the superman who, by the force of ruthless self-affirmation, rises above morality. He creates his own values; he does not submit to the values of others. If he has duties to others, it is only to other elite persons like himself.

Much more fundamental is Nietzsche's major thesis in the *Genealogy of Morals.* Here he contends that the whole tradition of moral philosophy, including the importance of the virtues, is a mask for the "will to power." There is not, and cannot be, any objective set of moral principles and virtues arrived at by reasoning that is always true; there is only a series of perspectives of what is right and good. Rather, as MacIntyre puts it, "Allegiance to such a view [of a unified, encyclopedic rationality] is always a sign of badness, of inadequately managed rancor and resentment. The conduct of life requires a rupture, a breaking down of such idols and a breaking up of fixed patterns so that something radically new can emerge."[9]

Articulating a response to Nietzsche and the other antivirtue moral theories is not our major enterprise. MacIntyre makes the attempt, so far as Nietzsche goes, with his powerful rejustification of the Aristotelian-Thomist tradition. But, as he himself admits, the gulf separating opposing fundamental moral theories is not convincingly closed by dialectic.[10] We will content ourselves with offering our view of medical ethics, in which virtues play an essential role, in the hope that what may not be convincing about virtue theories in the abstract may, in fact, be so when viewed within a practice with a definable telos like medicine.

The Contemporary Revival of Virtue

The recent revival of interest in the place of virtue in moral philosophy has inspired a set of new definitions. A few of these deserve mention to indicate the range of meanings, as well as the continuing evolution of the ancient conception.

Most influential is MacIntyre's definition in *After Virtue,* which, more than any other work, has given new life to virtue ethics. That book traces the degeneration of the classical tradition of virtue and indicates how the resulting loss of moral consensus has made moral discourse so difficult and frustrating. MacIntyre proposes that virtues be seen as dispositions or acquired qualities distinguished by the following characteristics: (1) they are necessary for humans to attain the goods internal to communal practices; (2) they sustain communal identities in which individuals can seek the good of their whole lives; and (3) they sustain traditions that provide practices and individual lives with necessary historical context. The elements of this definition telegraph MacIntyre's response to both the "encyclopedic" and the "genealogical" views of moral philosophy. They provide a "third way" between the encyclopedist's belief in a universal, unified set of rationally arrived-at truths, on the one hand, and, the multiple, historically determined, variant, and opposing perspectives of the genealogical view, on the other. That third way is argued in detail in MacIntyre's most recent book.[11]

Philippa Foot takes a functionalist view, identifying virtue as what is conducive to the individual's and the society's capacity to recognize the good and engage the will. Virtues are correctives to the tendency to act against the good.[12] Stanley Hauerwas takes a position close to MacIntyre's when he makes hope the formative element of the virtues whose soul is shared narrative and community.[13]

Pincoffs extends the moral sentiment theory of the British empiricists when he defines virtues as whatever makes us likable or affable to others. As a result, his list of virtues is so long that one wonders whether anything about us is not a virtue at some time, in some place, or under some circumstance. John Casey, in a recent provocative book entitled *Pagan Virtue*,[14] says that there is no "virtue" in virtue, since the virtues are determined and not the product of free wills. His view is akin to that of Edward Wilson, who contends that virtues may simply be genetically determined mechanisms to ensure survival of the gene pool.[15]

Finally, Carol Gilligan's proposal of a "different voice" in ethics offers a new insight into moral psychology pertinent to any definition of the virtues.[16] Her view is, in many ways, complementary to the classical view in that it suggests certain "humanistic" dispositions as virtues. Gilligan contends that these virtues are more consistent with the traditional moral psychology of women than that of men. The different voice is not limited to gender questions, but applies as well to modes of moral reasoning and behavior and to the hierarchy of moral values.

Conclusion

Given all the transitions in meaning and the diverging definitions of virtue, which concept shall we use in our inquiry into the place of the virtues in medical ethics? Without arguing the merits and demerits of each definition, we shall opt for the classical definitions of Aristotle and Thomas Aquinas. We do not think subsequent definitions have added anything to the essential notion, though some of them have enriched our understanding of its nuances. MacIntyre's application of the classical notion to practices within which we would include medicine is particularly helpful. The reasons for our choice will emerge as our argument unfolds, particularly in the teleological bent of our theory of medicine and medical ethics.

The history of the interrelationships between classical Greek philosophy, Stoical ethics, medieval thought, and modern ideas about ethics is fascinating. The differences and similarities in the concept of virtue, the good life, and the nature and destiny of man propounded by these world views shaped the concepts of virtue that emerged in the medieval and modern eras. Some of these interrelationships will become more apparent as we discuss the individual virtues of medicine in the chapters to follow.

As can be seen from our short sketch of the history of virtue theory, an enormous amount of development in virtue theory itself, as well as ethical theory in general, has occurred. Only in the last few years has a resurgence of interest in virtue theory occurred, as we have attempted in medical ethics to link principles, norms, and axioms, with the obvious clinical casuistry that is part of medical practice. W. Jaeger makes the point that Aristotle's doctrine of virtue as a mean may have come from Greek medicine. This doctrine too owes something to Plato's concept of health of body and soul as being a state of harmony and balance. Note also how often Aristotle used medicine as a model for his method and his ethics.[17] These comments suggest an important relationship between the ends of medicine and the virtues it requires of its practitioners, a point we will examine in Chapter 3.

It seems obvious that despite a proliferation of policies and guidelines, if the individual physician, as well as the patient, is not habitually disposed toward the good and generally to be trusted, terrible consequences occur in medicine and medical practice, from outright fraud to direct harm to patients. Our exploration of the link between the virtues and the qualities necessary for medical practice starts with the next chapter.

Objections to Virtue Theory in Medicine

Our proposal for relating virtue theory to medicine must face some of the serious objections to virtue theory applied to medicine that come from adherents of the four-principle approach, the latter largely proponents of deontological moral theory. In brief, how did we answer them?

That the virtues and traits of the specific practice of medicine are not immediately evident. Veatch has demonstrated that a wide variety of virtues have been promoted throughout history, some of which are repulsive to an adult, autonomy model of the patient–physician relation. Decisions about which virtues to emphasize are culture bound.[18] Thus virtue theory will tend to produce wrong conduct when the virtues it chooses are the wrong ones.

We answer this objection by targeting the major virtues that have been linked to the specific healing aim of medicine throughout its long history. Character traits influenced by culture occur, of course, but are not uncritically accepted, especially in the environment of increased self-criticism of medicine created by medical ethics today. Further, interpretations of the principles themselves are culturally driven, as are most moral senses we possess.[19] This objection does not in itself invalidate a virtue-theory approach.

Virtue theory is actually dangerous. Veatch's next objection is stronger: "Naked virtue together with the wrong virtues may well lead to wrong acts even though the intentions of the actor may be well-meaning."[20] This objection stems from the important insight that virtue theory cannot stand alone in a modern, pluralistic, secular society, since too much variability in the virtues to be emphasized might occur. Veatch is correct about this. For this reason, we take pains to argue and to demonstrate that virtue theory must be linked with the principles in an integrated medical ethics. Not only do we devote an early chapter to this linkup, but in each sketch of the virtues we examine how the virtues are linked with principles. For example, the virtue of justice has been combined with its principle; compassion, the virtue, with the principle of beneficence, and so on.

Then, too, none of the virtues stand in isolation. Veatch's argument depends a great deal on an example of a single virtue, benevolence. But the virtues, we argue, must all be linked with one another, not only through their definitions and the actions toward which they tend, but also with respect to *phronesis,* the act of practical intelligence that summates them and applies to particular situations.

Virtue theory is unnecessary in stranger medicine. Veatch's strongest objection comes from an argument that in an age of strangers, we need to be concerned about right conduct. In contrast, a *Gemeinschaft* in which we are all known to one another might possibly focus on the virtues of the individual healers and patients. Since Veatch argues that the virtues do not necessarily lead to right conduct, virtue theory is not needed in stranger medicine, the kind practiced in emergency rooms or by specialists largely unknown to patients. The latter physicians and other health professionals need to be guided by moral rules.[21] To this argument he adds further considerations about sectarian medicine and pluralism.

The answer to this objection is that right conduct cannot be guaranteed even by a principle approach. Indeed, without the virtues, there is no guarantee that one would be inclined to respect autonomy or the rules of informed consent. In an age of strangers, we need to be surer rather than less sure that the individuals who treat us are devoted to our good and that of the aim of medicine. We see Veatch's argument as actually strengthening the hand of virtue theory in medicine rather than weakening it. To our minds, secular pluralism can be overemphasized by deontologists and libertarians when it comes to medical practice. We offer a search for the enduring virtues of medicine as an alternative to efforts to find transcendent moral principles upon which to ground moral acts in medicine. Since so much change occurs in modern society, it is helpful to have both to guide us. As Tom Beauchamp notes in his thoughtful essay, "No duty-based theory need deny the importance of virtues and any viable theory of principles of duty, in my judgment, will include an account of virtue."[22] You can't have one without the other.

Training in virtues does not guarantee good results. This objection is a conflation of all the desolate reflections on how physicians in Germany could have been so supportive of Nazi initiatives, especially those of "biological purity." In a volume devoted to the Nuremberg Code, Elie Wiesel agonizes: "That doctors participated in the planning, execution, and justification of the concentration camp massacres is bad enough, but it went beyond medicine. Like the cancer of immorality, it spread into every area of spiritual, cultural, and intellectual endeavor. Thus, the meaning of what happened transcended its own immediate limits."[23] Wiesel writes of a famous Jewish professor, Shimon Dubnow, whose own student, Johann Siebert, not only taunted him in the ghetto but also eventually killed him. Wiesel states: "I couldn't understand these men who had, after all, studied for 8, 10, 12, or 14 years in German universities, which then were the best on the Continent, if not in the world. Why did their education not shield them from evil? This question haunted me."[24] The editors, Annas and Grodin, ask explicitly, "How could physician healers turn into murderers? This is among the most profound questions in medical ethics."[25]

The best answer to the question involves many different and complex factors.

Society itself was primed to develop a biological basis for its political platforms. The use of the best of the new science of genetics by the Nazis is well known. What is not as well known is that over half of all practicing physicians joined the Nazi party early on, even before Hitler came to power. The sad record is that many more than the forty-some physicians prosecuted in the Nuremberg trials participated in planning and carrying out the various programs that now have become so infamous. What is worse is that most of them, such as the euthanasia program, were justified by international practices, particularly by laws and procedures in the United States.[26] Part of the justification for sterilizing the retarded was to clean up the genes of the rest of the race, and part of the reason for euthanizing the demented was economic, a "preemptive triage," to free up beds needed for soldiers in the war effort.[27] But both of these initiatives against "worthless life" were based on published papers around the world in which similar proposals were being made, for example, in the *Journal of the American Psychiatric Association,* where killing the retarded, "nature's mistakes," was advocated.[28]

The lessons to be learned from this experience are that all individuals must be treated as ends in themselves, that the evils of wartime triage should not become ordinary or accepted ethical practices, and that a desire to practice modern, genetic-based health care will inevitably lead to efforts to "keep up" with the world literature, with standards of care elsewhere. Nazi physicians worried a lot about how the U.S. genetic laws were more advanced than theirs. A final point is this: Nazi physicians did not lose their sense of right and wrong. Their perception of the good was colored by society, mores, and their own craft and its standards at the time. The leading Nazi medical ethicist, Rudolf Ramm, echoing an earlier statement, said in 1942, "Only a good person can be a good physician."[29]

History can easily repeat itself. As the discussion of euthanasia and physician-assisted suicide escalates in the United States, and as the practices of abortion and euthanasia spread around the world, coupled with increased attention to genetic therapies, what is the "good" that will infuse the virtues in medical practice? We have focused on the goals of healing. But this is not enough to guarantee a good outcome, or even a consistent one, since one person's good is another's evil.

This is the reason that the virtues in medical practice must be coupled with a principle-based ethics. Further, neither one, nor the other, nor both conjoined, guarantee good behavior. Only critically reflective medical ethics and self-critical individuals of good character can offer some hope that history will not be repeated here. Science and medicine do not serve only external interests. They are also informed by and give credence to those interests. Our claim is only that a person of integrity, would be less likely to succumb to the fancies and foibles of any particular era.

Notes

1. See Giovanni Reale, *A History of Ancient Philosophy,* ed. and trans. by John R. Catan (Albany: State University of New York Press, 1987).
2. Justice for Aristotle, however, is the one virtue that admits of no extreme.

3. C. H. von Wright, *The Varieties of Goodness* (New York: Humanities Press, 1963).

4. Ludwig Edelstein, *Ancient Medicine: Selected Papers of Ludwig Edelstein,* ed. O. Temkin and C. L. Temkin (Baltimore, MD: Johns Hopkins University Press, 1967); see E. D. Pellegrino and A. A. Pellegrino, "Humanism and Ethics in Roman Medicine: Translation and Commentary on a Text of Scribonius Largus," *Literature and Medicine* 7 (1988):22–38.

5. See John M. Rist, *Stoic Philosophy* (London: Cambridge University Press, 1969), and Reale, *Ancient Philosophy.*

6. Immanuel Kant, *Grounding for the Metaphysics of Morals,* trans. James W. Ellington (Indianapolis, IN: Hackett Publishing Co., 1981), AK. 421, p. 30 and AK. 429, p. 36.

7. Ayn Rand, *The Virtue of Selfishness* (New York: New American Library, 1965).

8. H. Tristrum Engelhardt, Jr., and Michael Rie, "Morality for the Medical-Industrial Complex: A Code of Ethics for the Mass Marketing of Health Care," *New England Journal of Medicine* 319(16) (October 20, 1988):1086–1089.

9. Alasdair MacIntyre, *Three Rival Versions of Moral Enquiry: Encyclopedia, Geneology, and Tradition* (Notre Dame, IN: University of Notre Dame Press, 1990), p. 43.

10. Alasdair MacIntyre, *After Virtue,* 2d ed. (Notre Dame, IN.: Notre Dame University Press, 1984).

11. MacIntyre, *Three Rival Versions.*

12. Phillipa Foot, *"Virtues and Vices" and Other Essays in Moral Philosophy* (Berkeley: University of California Press, 1978).

13. Stanley Hauerwas, *Truthfulness and Tragedy: Further Investigations in Christian Ethics* (Notre Dame, IN: Notre Dame University Press, 1977).

14. John Casey, *Pagan Virtue* (New York: Oxford University Press, 1990).

15. Edward O. Wilson, *Sociobiology* (Cambridge, MA: Belknap/Harvard University Press, 1980).

16. Carol Gilligan, *In a Different Voice: Psychological Theory and Women's Development* (Cambridge, MA: Harvard University Press, 1982).

17. See Edmund D. Pellegrino, and David C. Thomasma, *A Philosophical Basis of Medical Practice* (New York: Oxford University Press, 1981), pp. 15–16, 82–99; Aristotle, *De Sensu,* in *The Works of Aristotle,* J. L. Beare tr., W. E. Ross ed. (New York: Oxford University Press, 1931), Ch. I, p. 436a; *Nichomachean Ethics,* viii, 1155a; *De Partibus Animalium,* I, 640a; *Rhetoric* I, c.1, 1355a–b.

18. Robert Veatch, "Against Virtue: A Deontological Critique of Virtue Theory in Medical Ethics," *Virtue in Medicine,* Vol. 17 of *The Philosophy and Medicine Series,* ed. Earl E. Shelp (Dordrecht/Boston: Reidel, 1985), pp. 334–337.

19. See the other essays in the volume just cited: Dietrich von Engelhardt, "Virtue and Medicine During the Enlightenment in Germany," in Shelp (ed.), *Virtue and Medicine,* pp. 63–80; Laurence B. McCullough, "Virtues, Etiquette, and Anglo-American Medical Ethics in the Eighteenth and Nineteenth Centuries," ibid., pp. 81–94; Marx W. Wartofsky, "Virtues and Vices: The Social and Historical Construction of Medical Norms," ibid., pp. 175–200.

20. Veatch, "Against Virtue," pp. 337–338.

21. Ibid., pp. 338–340.

22. Tom L. Beauchamp, "What's So Special About the Virtues?" in Shelp (ed.), *Virtue in Medicine,* p. 310.

23. Elie Weisel, "Preface," *The Nazi Doctors and the Nuremberg Code,* ed. George J. Annas and Michael A. Grodin (New York: Oxford University Press, 1992), p. vii.

24. Ibid.

25. Annas and Grodin, "Introduction," *The Nazi Doctors and the Nuremberg Code*, p. 3.

26. Robert Proctor, "Nazi Doctors, Racial Medicine, and Human Experimentation," *The Nazi Doctors and the Nuremberg Code*, pp. 17–31.

27. Ibid., p. 24.

28. Ibid.

29. As quoted at the head of Proctor, "Nazi Doctors, Racial Medicine, and Human Experimentation," *The Nazi Doctors and the Nuremberg Code*, p. 17.

2

The Link Between Virtues, Principles, and Duties

Although it remained the central concept in ethics for so long, and although it is now being refurbished, there are certain limitations to any ethical system based solely on virtue. One such limitation, as the preceding chapter shows, is the variety of definitions of virtue and of the virtues in different philosophical systems. To unravel or reconcile these differences is a formidable task, requiring nothing less than a reconciliation of opposing philosophical systems. MacIntyre has recently shown how difficult—perhaps impossible—such an enterprise must be, since so many of the differences are, to use his terminology, "incommensurable and untranslatable."[1]

There is in our pluralistic society no agreed-upon philosophical anthropology or metaphysics. Lacking these, we lose the foundation upon which some common idea of the good for humans could be based. As a result, the telos toward which the virtues were thought to dispose the agent becomes vague. Differences in moral ends, as a consequence, become relativized, subjective, and negotiable in response to the exigencies of the moment. As a further consequence, the virtues ordered to those ends of necessity become problematic.

But even where there might be agreement on a definition of the good, there is a certain circularity in the logic of virtue ethics. The morally good act is one done by the virtuous person; the virtuous person is one who performs morally good acts. This circular reasoning is tolerable when some common notion of the good is accepted by all. When there is no such common notion, the logical consistency of the connections between character and morally good acts is no longer sustainable. Some justification for either character or acts must be sought beyond virtue. The need for specific moral action guides becomes acute. To counter the inevitable resultant pull to moral subjectivism and emotivism, which an absence of action guides invites, thinkers turn to principles as the grounding of ethics.

Principles are general or universal guides to action. They may be derived from more fundamental moral postulates and intuitions or accepted as prima facie moral truths that should be respected unless there is a morally compelling reason not to do so. Examples of principles derived from more fundamental a priori moral concepts are Kant's categorical imperative, Mill and Bentham's principle of utility, or the Scholastic principle of synderesis—do good and avoid evil. Examples of prima facie principles are those proposed by W. D. Ross.[2] Ross' method is employed by Beauchamp and Childress in their highly influential *Principles of Biomedical Ethics.*"[3]

Our view in this book is that virtue-based ethics is not, by itself, a sufficient foundation for medical ethics, given the complexities of this subject today. But neither is it expendable, since the character of the physician (and, of course, of the patient) is still at the heart of moral choice and action. It is the agent who interprets principles, selects the ones to apply or ignore, puts them in an order of priority, and shapes them in accord with his life history and current life situations. This reality has been too often ignored in past biomedical and clinical ethics explorations. A proper balance must be struck between rule-based and virtue-based ethics for the health of both.

Principle-based ethics has its own limitations. Indeed, in recognition of these limitations, we are currently in the midst of a backlash against "principlism" in medical ethics.[4] Some say that principles are too abstract, that their use in moral judgments is too formularized and far removed from the concrete human particulars of moral choice. Others decry their lack of grounding in the great moral traditions. Still others have found principles too much dominated by the moral psychology of white males of European extraction and thus meaningless to women, non-Europeans, or "right brain" (analytical) as against "left brain" (intuitive/affective) thinkers.

Remedies for the perceived defects of principle-based ethics have been sought in a variety of new approaches. Attention has turned to other sources of morality or, at the very least, to other methods of moral analysis. One alternative is a more sophisticated modern version of casuistry as advanced by Toulmin, Jonsen, Hauerwas, Prody, Hunter, and, to a certain extent, MacIntyre. These writers emphasize the narratives, stories, or traditions of peoples and individuals. Moral acts are then judged in terms of the values of the communities within which moral agents live and thrive. Reich appeals for an "experiential ethic," which, as we understand it, is a psychologically attentive ethic whose application he illustrates in difficult cases involving disabled newborns. Others find the major remedy for the defects of principle-based ethics in an alternate ethic inherent in feminine psychology.[5] Finally, for some, a hermeneutic approach that reads the medical relationship as a text is the preferred remedy.[6]

These alternatives to principle-based ethics have certain similarities to virtue ethics, since they place more emphasis on persons, agents, and circumstances than principles do. But we think they cannot stand alone any more than virtue ethics can. Whether built on experience, differences in moral psychology, casuistry, narrative, or textual approach, these alternatives tend ultimately to subjectivism, psychologism, and emotivism. Our experiences are necessarily limited; our "stories" are culture bound, as are our traditions; our analysis of particular cases runs the constant danger of "situationism"; and a gender-based ethic has its own kind of insulation. This is not to deny that each of these new approaches has something to contribute to medical ethics and must be taken into account in any attempt at an integral or comprehensive moral philosophy of medicine.

It is our contention that virtue-based ethics, as well as the newer alternatives to principle-based ethics, must somehow be joined to principle-based ethics if the limitations of each approach are to be balanced by the strengths of the other. We will not attempt to argue the superiority of a virtue-based ethic over the more recent alternatives to principles. We believe that as we spell out more clearly the relationship between principles and virtues, and apply that relationship to the individual virtues in the medical relationship, many of the nuances of the alternatives to principle-based ethics can be accommodated.

Is There a Link Between Virtues and Principles?

In virtue-based ethics, virtue is usually contrasted with duty-based or principle-based systems. The possibility of linkages between them is not often emphasized. Kant "solves" the problem by conflating virtue and duty; he defines the virtuous person as one who does his or her duty, who acts in conformity with the supreme moral principle of ethics: the categorical imperative. Beauchamp and Childress, like Frankena, attempt linkages by relating certain virtues with certain prima facie principles.

Neither of these solutions is satisfying. Kant robs principles, duty, and virtue of their distinctiveness, condensing the whole into a rationalistic enterprise that leaves no room for the Aristotelian-Thomist notion of habitus or dispositions that predispose to right and good action and character. Beauchamp and Childress keep the notions of principles and virtues separate but do not provide a conceptually convincing way to link them or differentiate them. MacIntyre has done more than any contemporary ethicist, with the possible exception of Elizabeth Anscombe, to define virtue in terms of practices and the communities in which those practices are embodied. But he has not yet put virtues into any clear conceptual relationship with principles or duties.

These difficulties notwithstanding, moral theory is the poorer for want of a satisfactory way to integrate virtue and principle in moral analysis and decision making. Is the virtuous person simply one who uses principles rightly, who reasons correctly and develops tight, convincing arguments based on principles? Manifestly, this cannot be the case. One may master the techniques of moral analysis and yet be a person of dubious character—something not so rare as one might hope among skilled ethicists. Moreover, as the Minor Hippias so poignantly illustrates, one may develop substantial and skillful arguments leading to conclusions that no person of good character can accept.[7] Conversely, we know many good people who we would trust to act well under most circumstances, but who are ignorant of ethical principles and might not be able to articulate cogent reasons for their choices. Ethics is clearly more than a technical exercise in moral decision analysis.

We face an important dilemma here for any virtue theory: on the one hand, one may have a good grasp of ethical principles and yet not apply them correctly or in a dependable way; on the other hand, there are persons of character who may not be aware of moral principles or may even reason incorrectly about them, but are of such character that they can be depended upon to act rightly. Is it sufficient to settle for character alone, then, as a basis for ethics? Is virtue sufficient for all occasions in moral philosophy?

This cannot be the case, since good dispositions or good character alone will not ensure that the act or moral choice is good. It can ensure good intentions and motives. But the moral quality of acts and persons depends upon the way intentions, circumstances, and acts relate to each other. Moral principles are the benchmarks against which we may assess the moral quality of these relationships. A complete moral theory must, at a minimum, tie some conceptual knots between duty, principles, and virtue.

Medicine, as we will argue in the next chapter, is at its heart a moral enterprise. The principles of medical ethics are statements of the right and good that derive from the ends and purposes of medical activity—healing, helping, and caring in a special kind of human relationship. The duties of doctors are the obligations voluntarily assumed by those who engage in the activity of medicine and who, in consequence, commit themselves to the ends of medicine. They are also committed ipso facto to the principles that must guide medical actions if its ends are to be realized. Virtues are the traits of character that dispose the agent—the doctor and the patient—to choices that will attain those ends. Virtues, in one sense, confer the powers (*virtus*) to make moral choices such that they are always or *ut in pluribus*[8] oriented to the proper ends of medicine. The person of character or virtue intends habitually to pursue the ends of the activity in question. It is her design, her *ratio agibilium,*[9] her reason for acting both as to ends and means. Aquinas used *recta ratio agibilium*[10] as his definition of prudence—a right reason in acting. Is virtue then simply a proper moral sense, as Hume and the British empiricists would have it? Moral sense as an intuition of what is good is surely part of the idea of virtue, but not the whole of it because there is also a rational component in virtue. Phronesis, or prudence, is both a moral and an intellectual virtue that disposes one habitually to choose the right thing to do in a concrete moral situation.

In morals, a principle is the most fundamental and most universalizable moral entity. It is a guide to action binding in all circumstances for deontologists, or at least in a prima facie way for those whose deontology allows for some exceptions. A principle is derived from the consideration of moral action in its most fundamental aspects. It is often perceived intuitively like the most fundamental of moral principles, for example, the principle of synderesis in scholastic thought—do good and avoid evil. Because of their generality, principles need to be interpreted in their application to particular cases. We note here with Hare that universalizability and generality are not the same.[11] Some moral principles are quite specific and still universalizable.

A principle is a statement of some fundamental and universal moral truth that is also expressible as an action guide. Thus, it is a principle to state that humans *qua* humans are owed respect for their ability to make reasoned choices that are their own and that others may or may not share. This principle is fundamental in the sense that it is grounded in the fact of being human, a species of being that is essentially defined in part by its capability to reason, to plan for the future, and thus to provide self-direction. To violate this capacity for self-governance without the gravest reasons is a grave deprivation of another person of his humanity. Only the gravest reasons—loss of the capacity for self-governance by brain dysfunction, for example, or the use of self-governance of another—could justify relaxation or overriding of this principle.

Stated as a moral action guide, this respect for the power of self-governance enjoins that we act so that we respect, enhance, or empower those with whom we interact to realize the ends they choose for a single action, a series of actions, or their whole lives. Whether these acts are morally neutral, right, and good, or wrong and bad, depends upon their congruence with the ends or purposes of human life. We presume, as Aquinas did, that the ends individual persons choose are chosen under the appearance of good.[12]

The virtuous person is virtuous with respect to this principle not simply because she observes the principle, but because she has not initialized it, made it synonymous with her intentions with respect to other humans, is habitually disposed to respect that principle, and is disposed to do so excellently—that is, as fully as possible. Thus, the virtuous person is not virtuous because she respects the principle, but because she recognizes the fundamental and universal nature of this principle, sees it not just as a duty in the Kantian sense, but as part of her character—incised, so as to speak, in the etymological sense of the word "character," into her very person and identity. The virtuous person cultivates *areté* in the way she actualizes the virtue in her moral choices and actions.

The principle, however,—whether it is respect for self-governance, benevolence, justice, honesty, truth telling, and so on—is not morally meritorious because it is respected by the virtuous person. Rather, we respect the virtuous person because he is someone we know and can trust will practice the virtue in question with perfection-seeking diligence. This pursuit of perfection in the practice of the virtue will be most evident at what we shall call the "moral margin"—that large domain of choices and actions where the contrasts between right and good, wrong and bad, are not starkly obvious, where virtue and vice merge into the morally neutral and where those who pursue duty strictly *qua* duty do not feel impelled to go beyond the literal letter of the moral law.

Similarly, a virtuous person is not virtuous because her actions are judged admirable by those around her, as Hume might contend. Rather, we deem a person virtuous because she does perceive, and act, habitually in a way that exhibits the habitual disposition to perfection that, as humans, we perceive to be consistent with what it is to be a good person.

In Chapter 13 we will distinguish between this construal of virtue and supererogation and show, in some common practical moral choices facing the health profession today, how virtue-based ethics makes a difference.

Principles, then, are general statements of what guides the actions of a good person. A person is not virtuous because he follows the principle or does his duty, as Kant would have it. Rather, the principle derives its validity from the moral relationship that should obtain between rational beings capable of choosing their own values, ends, purposes, and life plans. The virtuous person, in possession of phronesis, has the necessary intellectual capacity to discern what is right and good in a particular case. His actions grow out of practical wisdom and are generalizable. It is prudence, phronesis, or practical wisdom that helps us recognize the good and the right. All humans possess the tendency to do good and avoid evil. Further, they possess a natural habit of the mind (Syncleresis) that enables knowledge of practical principles. They differ among themselves in their definitions of what is good, both in general and in particular, and in the degree to which they deem their actions accord with the good morally requisite. The vicious person does evil under the semblance of good. In the preceding chapter, we noted antivirtue theorists such as Macchiavelli, Nietzsche, and, in the philosophy of medicine, Engelhardt. Even these thinkers, who confuse virtues and vices, still retain a basic belief in the idea of virtue. A principle, then, codifies and provides the rule of predictability of the good person—what we can expect him to do in a particular situation. The popular parlor game Scruples builds on that very predictability. Even if one argues that there is no need for the virtues, since all they represent is a strict adherence to a rule, the inner disposition or "virtue" would be toward excellence in obedience or subservience to the rule.

In making any moral choice or selecting an action, principles are necessary as benchmarks, but they are not sufficient, since every moral act is a particular act embedded in time, space, place, and persons. A moral decision is not a decision about a principle, but about the relationship of circumstances, intentions, and ends to a principle. Moralists recognize the infinite diversity of particulars in any moral act. They know the principles and may order them in relation to the particulars and facts. They do so formally. Most of us, moralists included, in our individual decisions do so less formally. The virtue of prudence, that is, practical wisdom, enables us to arrive at the right and good ordering of principles and concrete facts in particular cases. Nowhere is this truer than in medical decisions, since each person's experience of illness is unique and its relationship to moral principle is far from indisputably evident. The prudent physician or patient is the one who can order habitually fact and principle most sensitively and correctly to each other and act appropriately to achieve the good for the patient—and, parenthetically, for the physician at work.

It is important at this juncture to distinguish between two senses in which we may speak of personal morality—one sense of which is perilous, the other essential. If by personal morality we mean—as so many contemporary moralists do—that morality is a personal, idiosyncratic matter in which each of us makes what, for ourselves, is a right and good decision, and that our personal imprint confers moral legitimacy, then such a conception would destroy any idea of principle—except the principle of moral egotism. However, personal morality may also refer to the person as central to moral decisions, as an agent, as a bearer of a unique experience that must be brought into some alignment with something beyond the person—the principles of morality. This construal of the personal is a necessity if ethics is to be more than a chess game with formulaic responses to opening gambits dictated by principles irrespective of circumstances, intentions, or ends.

Aquinas cogently argues that moral quality—and culpability as well—rests in the ordering of principles and concrete lived realities at the moment of moral choice and action.[13] Moral acts are inextricably tied to the who, what, where, how, and why of our personal lives. We are saved from the errors of situationist, emotivist, and egoist ethics by principles. But, by themselves, the principles can depersonalize and dehumanize. Virtue-based ethics link principles and obligations as abstract entities to the circumstances of our personal lives through the virtue of prudence.[14] Aquinas returned the notion of the good to its central position in the moral life, adding what Aristotle and Plato lacked: a clear notion of the ultimate good, the *summum bonum*, that is, union with God. In Aquinas' view, virtues dispose us to attain the supreme good, and specific duties are measured in terms of their congruence with virtuous behavior.

Duties are specific statements of what is required or morally obliged, either by some principle or rule, in contrast to what we might wish to do. The founders of moral philosophy—Socrates, Plato, and Aristotle—were more concerned with the good and the virtues, those traits that habitually dispose the moral agent to the good. It was the Stoics who introduced the idea that it was the duty of humans to live virtuously, the virtues themselves being defined in terms of congruence with the immutable laws of nature. Christian and Jewish thought often took the same turn, requiring a life in conformity with the supreme law of God as enunciated in Revelation. Kant went furthest in equating duty with principle. For him, the supreme logic of duty was contained in the categorical imperative revealed to humans intuitively by the rational will.

Hume defined a virtue as a "quality of the mind agreeable to or approved by every one, who considered or contemplates it."[15] Thus, virtues are those traits that evoke a sentiment of approbation in others. Hume, moreover, imputed virtue to motives from which acts emanate rather than to the acts themselves: "We must look within to find the moral quality. This we cannot do directly and, therefore, we fix our attention on actions as on external signs. . . . The ultimate object of praise and approbation is the motive that produced them [the acts]."[16] This comes close to Abailard's location of moral quality in the quality of our intentions. Hume's view of virtues based on social approbation is the best articulated of the naturalist theories that grounded duty as well as virtue in social custom, education, or other accidentals of our situation in life and our individual biographies. Duty, in this view, is the obligation to act in conformity with what is socially approved, inculcated, or accepted as convention. The moral principle, in this view, would be: "So act that the motive behind your action is one that will be universally approved or is congruent with social convention." This has been called "virtue by consensus." It is a view shared by Hume, Hutcheson, and Adam Smith. V. M. Hope shows, in his interesting study, that these authors may differ in what they consider morally appropriate and in what constitutes consensus.[17]

Beauchamp and Childress, the most influential of today's principle-based theorists of biomedical ethics, link virtue, rule, and principle through motivation— very much like Hume. They opine that "to be virtuous is not only to be disposed to bring about a good state of affairs, but also to desire what is good."[18] Unfortunately, they do not provide as full a treatment of what constitutes the "good" as we think necessary. It is possible to be disposed to do what is right, to intend to do it, and to do it while desiring to be able to avoid doing it."[19] We would interpret Beauchamp and Childress to mean that the virtuous physician would seek the good of the patient as the proper end of medicine. His motive should be primarily to fulfill that end—not to gain the fee, prestige, power, or preferment.

Beauchamp and Childress hold that principle, obligation-based ethics, and virtue-based ethics are compatible and complement each other. A virtue-based ethic is insufficient by itself because it provides no action guide to help even in deciding how to confront especially difficult dilemmas. This position makes sense. Beauchamp and Childress propose that for every principle there is a corresponding virtue.[20] As one reviews their table,[21] however, the "correspondence or correlation" they propose seems somewhat contrived. Thus, the principle of respect for autonomy becomes the virtue of respectfulness, nonmaleficence becomes the virtue of nonmalevolence, beneficence becomes benevolence, justice remains as justice, verity is truthfulness, and so on. The correspondence seems to consist largely in converting the action guides to subjective states and renaming them, but establishing no essential difference between them.

In the case of what they call "derivative obligations" and "ideals of action," the same words are used for the corresponding virtues. Beauchamp and Childress admit that three of the four cardinal virtues—prudence, courage, and temperance—do not fit their schema. They conclude that the relations between obligations and virtues are "not tidy," but "no theory should seek tidiness at the expense of comprehensiveness."[22]

We agree with the general conclusion that virtue and duty-based theories complement each other. Each does provide a different and complementary perspective on moral choice and action. But we maintain, especially in the confines of medical ethics, that a more precise conceptual linkage is desirable. For example, Beauchamp and Childress classify compassion as an "ideal of action." They consider it desirable but not morally obligatory in the same way that respect for autonomy is morally obligatory.

But let us examine several of the "medical" virtues in the medical relationship a little more closely. We take **compassion**, for example, as a virtue of special importance in the medical relationship. We define compassion as the capacity of physicians to feel something of the unique predicament of the patient, to enter into the patient's experience of illness and, as a result, to suffer vicariously the patient's anxiety, pain, fear (and so on). We will explore this virtue in more detail in Chapter 6. We take compassion as a virtue necessary to the ends of medicine as we describe them in the next chapter. In our view, the doctor cannot heal unless he makes his objective judgments of what ought to be done medically congruent with what the patient perceives ought to be done. The patient's sense of "ought" will be defined by what he, the patient thinks worthwhile, that is, the things that give a unique identity to his life at the moment in time when the doctor advises what is medically indicated. Without compassion, only objective medical good, the lowest order of patient good, is obtainable.[23] For fuller healing, the objective assessment of medical or technical good must be modulated by compassion. By necessity, in achieving the ends of medicine, compassion must be a virtue of the good physician. Although it is an internal disposition, compassion is also manifest in the physician's behavior.

Intellectual honesty is a somewhat different example. It can be required as a duty in conformity with a moral action guide—that is, "always disclose accurately to your patient and colleagues the extent of your knowledge and ignorance." Intellectual honesty can, in part at least, be assessed from our actions alone. Yet we could not be honest unless we possessed the virtue of honesty, the habitual disposition not to deceive, or to move positively to reveal what we know and do not know about the clinical situation—the diagnosis, treatment, prognosis, and so on.

Benevolence is a virtue that need not necessarily be linked to beneficence. One might wish to harm a patient whom one does not like, who has not paid his bill, who is abusive, or who is physically threatening. The doctor could act beneficiently toward such a patient because of fear of retribution, a lawsuit, or loss of reputation— none of them worthy motives. The virtue of benevolence would be absent but the principle of beneficence would nonetheless be respected, at least in the objective sense. The same might apply to respect for persons, justice, temperance, and so on. We think less of the physician who lacks these virtues even if his acts conform objectively to moral principles and the duties the principle entails. The importance of virtue, as Beauchamp and Childress suggest, is that in any given case, the virtuous physician is more likely to act according to right principles. And, we would add, the virtuous physician will strive for excellence, for fulfillment of the full implications of the spirit of the principle. Thus the virtuous physician is one who can be trusted to act rightly in whatever circumstance he encounters. If the physician has the master virtue of prudence, she can more rightly adjust the deeper and genuine meaning of principles to the particularities of the case in question by seeing more clearly what compassion, wisdom, courage, and justice require in this case and in these circumstances.

A truly satisfying conceptual linkage between virtues and principles is difficult to discern. But we also know that we want a physician who is virtuous in the sense of possessing the virtues specific to achieving the ends of medicine. This is a sufficient warrant to educate physicians in virtue, as well as in principle and duty.

A Formal Linkage of Virtues and Principles

One of us (Thomasma) with Graber has explored the relationship between the virtues and moral theory,[24] distinguishing three ways in which virtues and theory can be linked: (1) "tacked on" after the fact, (2) by mediation, and (3) by substitution.

In the first view, proposed by many thinkers, Pence among them, we first determine the moral rightness of an act, using one or another of several moral theories or modes of analysis. After this, the work of the moral philosopher is probably completed.[25] Then the work of educators, trainers, politicians, psychologists, behaviorists, and others begins, with attempts to "instill" the desire or motivation to accomplish the moral activity. Examples of instilling motivation are almost always external: by passing laws, offering incentives, and the like. A good example can be found in the country of Singapore. In order to move from a poor agrarian society thirty years ago to a modern city-state today, laws were passed to train the populace in the smooth running of a society. To discourage urinating in elevators, as one example, as soon as ammonia from the urine is detected, the elevator locks, a hidden camera turns on and records the event, an alarm rings in the Housing and Development Board, and the police are dispatched to apprehend the culprit. The individual gets a big fine, and his picture may find its way into the newspaper.[26] Not all examples of external motivation are so extreme. The rules about obtaining informed consent from individuals in medical research are more modest but just as far-reaching.

A second method of relating the virtues to principles and their theories is mediation. In this view, when conflicts among principles occur, the virtuous person is able to mediate between them, or find a way to apply them, through internalization of the good as proposed by those principles. Henry Beecher argued the following about human experimentation:

> Rules will not curb the unscrupulous . . . the best approach concerns the character, wisdom, experience, honesty, imaginativeness and sense of responsibility of the investigator who, in all cases of doubt or where serious consequences might remotely occur, will call in his peers and get the benefit of their counsel.[27]

Franz Ingelfinger, once editor of *The New England Journal of Medicine,* opined in a famous article written near the end of his life that if the medical professional does not have the requisite virtues to internalize objective rules and standards, then they will not be carried out.[28]

Along these lines, Bernard Lonergan notes how the appropriation of any truth occurs in both the cognitive and the volitional realms. "To appropriate a truth is to make it one's own."[29] But since reasonableness demands that we link what we think and what we do (otherwise, a psychological disjunction occurs), there is a "volitional appropriation of truth that consists in our willingness to live up to it." Thereafter, there is also a "sensitive appropriation of truth that consists in an adaptation of our sensibility to the requirements of our knowledge and our decisions."[30] Following this insight, Lonergan notes that learning is identification of oneself with the truth, and orientation of the self to the "palpable environment," as he calls it.[31]

The third method of relating virtues and principles is substitution. In this view, internalization of the truth has occurred to such an extent that the principles and rules no longer need to exist. This would characterize the Singaporean who would never think of urinating in an elevator! More to the point, substitution entails such a complete internalization of the virtues that no rules, guidelines, regulations, and the like would be necessary in society. It represents the idealized world longed for by Beecher in his assessment of what is needed in institutions that do human subject research.

As we have already argued, however, virtue cannot substitute for moral principles. One reason is that virtues can impel us to right and good acts only generally and for the most part (St. Thomas called this an ethical certitude, *ut in pluribus*).[32] Another way of putting this is that there is no metaphysical certitude in moral matters. So the second reason virtue cannot substitute for moral principles is that human experience demonstrates all too well that not all human beings are at the same level of moral development. National guidelines, public moral policy, and moral rules are necessary to establish a minimum expectation of everyone. This is especially important in health care, where so much care involves strangers who do not know one another, much less one another's values.

These reflections offer a clue to the formal linkage of the virtues and principles. Just as ethical principles function in many different ways, not only within a specific moral theory in which they are embodied but also with respect to their application, so to do the virtues function in many different ways within a life experience and a network of such experiences that we have called a "moral community." Principles can be used by individuals and societies to command action, to assess actions, to evaluate actions, and so on. Virtues likewise have many different relationships. That is why MacIntyre underlines the interrelationships of virtues and principles when he notes:

> Rules and virtues are interrelated. To possess the virtue of justice, for example, involves both a will to give to each person what is due to him or her and a knowledge of how to apply the rules which prevent violations of that order in which each receives his or her due. To understand the application of rules as part of the exercise of the virtues is to understand the point of rule-following, just because one cannot understand the exercise of the virtues except in terms of their role in constituting the type of life in which alone the human *telos* is to be achieved.[33]

From the point of view of **the affective and emotional life**, the virtues are incrementally more powerful dispositions to strike a balance between two extremes. Using the example of compassion from our earlier discussion in this chapter, compassion would allow the physician to achieve a balance between the extremes of withdrawal from the patient's plight, on the one hand, and overengagement in the patient's life, on the other.

From the point of view of **the agent**, the virtues could represent a choice to act in a certain way in given circumstances. Lonergan analyzed how a decision to adopt a truth involves not only a cognitive but also a volitional component. It is this latter component that we honor in a virtuous person when rewards are passed out. Usually these are public displays of our acknowledgment that the individual did not have to choose to spend time each year working for the Symphony Benefit Ball, but did so despite a busy schedule because of her commitment to the good life of the community.

Our discussion of intention in the previous section now comes into play. The agent bonds with the good or the right thing proposed in the principle in an internal way, so that increasingly, through training, habit, and eventually conscious choice, his behavior is molded by the right and the good. Not only is this satisfying when one's mind and heart move in the same direction, but also it is fulfilling in a way that confirms our nature as moral beings.

From the point of view of **the action that is done**, the virtues can be seen as applications of the moral rule or principle to individual circumstances. What is finally achieved is a prudential judgment about the circumstances, an interpretative act that requires that all the virtues be unified in the person toward an end. Our discussion of phronesis in medical practice will consider this unifying feature in more detail.

Formally speaking, however, the virtues are conditions of possibility for the implementation of principles and moral rules. This is the essential linkage hinted at by Ingelfinger's intuition that, without the virtuous agent, no amount of rule making will ever change the behavior of individuals. Simply put, internalization of the right and the good through training and disposition will not only ensure application of the meaning of moral rules to life circumstances, but will also lead to refinements of the moral principles, and even to new moral theories that will try to resolve the new issues of the day.

This is also the reason why developments occur in any discipline, not just in ethics, and why one cannot easily shift from one sphere of moral inquiry to another, as MacIntyre has so eloquently argued. There is a fundamental formal tie-in of the principles, both to and from the life experiences of individuals in moral communities.

We would hold that this does not automatically lead to a conclusion that the life world of experience relativizes and enculturates moral rules to such an extent that they cannot be understood or applied outside of the environment that shaped them. But it does mean that intense labor must be involved to extrapolate their essence for use in this way, just as intense effort must be made to ascertain if there are indeed inherent human propensities, inclinations, disinclinations, that transcend history and culture. Movement in both directions, toward the universal moral rules and toward a universal human nature, will always be problematic from the point of view of the formal linkage of virtues with principles.

Conclusion

In the long run, whether or not a conceptual link can be established between principle, duty, and virtue is not as important as recognition that the character of the physician is an irreducible factor in the healing relationship. How he or she interprets the moral principles, selects the values that will predominate, and shape self-interest will be more important than how the moral principles are formulated and described. As Oakeshott puts it, all morality is a matter *inter homines*—a matter of relationships between persons[34]—not a chess game pitting principles and rules against each other.

This irreducibility of the character of the moral agent, the physician in medical ethics, is a fact, regardless of the model of ethical reasoning one elects—principle- or rule-based, duty-based, casuistic, situational, emotivist, egoistic, intuitionist, and so on. In every ethical theory there comes a moment of opportunity, the use of the theory by a particular person in a particular circumstance. In that moment, the virtues will make the difference, making a good theory better in ameliorating the harm of erroneous theories.

Notes

1. Alasdair MacIntyre, *After Virtue,* 2d ed. (Notre Dame, IN: Notre Dame University Press, 1984), pp. 190–195.

2. W. D. Ross, *The Right and the Good* (Indianapolis: Hackett, 1988).

3. Tom L. Beauchamp and James F. Childress, *Principles of Biomedical Ethics,* 3d ed. (New York: Oxford University Press, 1989).

4. See the *Journal of Medicine and Philosophy* 15(2) (April 1990).

5. Nel Noddings, *Caring: A Feminine Approach to Ethics and Moral Education* (Berkeley: University of California Press, 1984).

6. See Stephen L. Daniel (Guest Ed.), "Interpretation in Medicine," *Theoretical Medicine* 11 (1) (March, 1990), entire issue.

7. Plato, *Lesser Hippias* in *The Dialogues of Plato,* trans. B. Jowett, intro. by Raphael Demos (New York: Random House, 1937), pp. 715–729.

8. Generally, for the most part true. Ethical principles before the age of reason were not considered to be true with metaphysical, but rather with ethical, certitude. Exception were admitted in principle. See MacIntyre, *After Virtue.*

9. St. Thomas Aquinas, *Summa Theologiae,* 2, 2ae, qq. 47–48.

10. St. Thomas Aquinas, *Summa Theologiae,* 1, 2ae, q. 57, a. 4.

11. R. M. Hare, *Freedom and Reason* (New York: Oxford-Clarendon Press, 1985), pp. 3–37.

12. St. Thomas Aquinas, *Summa Theologiae,* 1, 2ae, qq. 9–10; q. 18.

13. *Ibid,* qq. 55–67; 2, 2ae, qq. 47–51.

14. Etienne Gilson, *Moral Values and the Moral Life: The Ethical Theory of St. Thomas Aquinas* (Hamden, CT: Shoe String Press, 1961).

15. David Hume, *An Enquiry Concerning the Principles of Morals,* ed. J. B. Schneewind (Indianapolis: Hackett, 1988), p. 68, n. 50.

16. David Hume, *A Treatise of Human Nature,* ed. L. A. Selby-Bigge (New York: Oxford-Clarendon Press, 1978), p. 477.

17. V. M. Hope, *Virtue by Consensus: The Moral Philosophy of Hutcheson, Hume and Adam Smith* (New York: Oxford-Clarendon Press, 1989), p. 2.

18. Beauchamp and Childress, *Principles,* p. 375.

19. Ibid.

20. Ibid., p. 379.

21. Ibid., p. 380.

22. Ibid., p. 381

23. Pellegrino and Thomasma, *For the Patient's Good: Toward the Restoration of Beneficence in Health Care* (New York: Oxford University Press, 1988).

24. Glenn C. Graber and David C. Thomasma, *Theory and Practice in Medical Ethics* (New York: Continuum, 1989), pp. 151–172.

25. Gregory Pence, *Ethical Options in Medicine* (Oradell, N.J.: Medical Economics, 1980), pp. 17ff.

26. Stan Sesser, "A Reporter at Large: A Nation of Contradictions," *The New Yorker* 67(47) (January 13, 1992):37–68, n. 54.

27. Henry K. Beecher, "Tentative Statement Outlining the Philosophy and Ethical Principles Governing the Conduct of Research on Human Beings at the Harvard Medical School," *Experimentation with Human Beings,* ed. Jay Katz (New York: Russell Sage Foundation, 1972), p. 848.

28. Franz Ingelfinger, "Arrogance," *New England Journal of Medicine* 303(26) (December, 25 1980):1507–1511.

29. Bernard Lonergan, *Insight: A Study of Human Understanding* (San Francisco: Harper & Row, 1978), p. 558.

30. Ibid.

31. Ibid., p. 559.

32. See note 8.

33. Alasdair MacIntyre, *Three Rival Versions, of Moral Enquiry: Encyclopedia, Geneology, and Tradition* (Notre Dame, IN: University of Notre Dame Press, 1990), p. 139.

34. Michael Oakeshott, *"Rationalism in Politics" and Other Essays* (Indianapolis: Liberty Press, 1991), p. 295.

3

Medicine as a Moral Community

The moral life is a life *inter homines*.
MICHAEL OAKESHOTT[1]

Alasdair MacIntyre has stressed repeatedly that the interrelationship of ethical virtues and principles relies upon the grounding of both in the community and its values. As he says of the community and moral rules:

> Detach them [the moral rules] from their place in defining and constituting a whole way of life and they become nothing but a set of arbitrary prohibitions, as they too often became in later periods. To progress in both moral enquiry and the moral life is then to progress in understanding *all* the various aspects of that life, rules, precepts, virtues, passions, actions as parts of a single whole.[2]

It is therefore important in our line of argument to consider the ways in which medicine itself functions as the moral community that both shapes the ends of the moral life of those who practice health care healing and the means by which these ends emerge in their virtuous actions.

Challenges in Professional Ethics

The most crucial dilemmas of medical ethics today are not those arising from medicine's scientific progress. They are dilemmas of professional ethics, those that go to the heart of what it is to be a physician. In these matters, medicine faces an unenviable choice. It must reconcile two opposing orders—one based on the primacy of its covenant with patients and the other based on the ethos of self-interest. Think for a moment of the major challenges to this tension between self-interest and altruism: whether to disclose one's HIV-positive status, having an economic interest in an MRI unit to which one refers patients, whether there is a duty to treat all patients who request care, the problem of health care for the poor and one's obligations in this regard, the reform of the health care system, conflicts about requests or public policy for physician-assisted suicide, integrity in scientific research, the medical-industrial complex, physicians' incentives as gatekeepers to keep costs down, and many others. Each of these dilemmas, although occasioned by technology, arises from changing roles of the profession in response to public and private expectations. Something of the past is inevitably lost, not always for the worse. But the profession is placed at risk too.

Should the health professions, as some prominent medical ethicists are urging, reshape our ethical codes to conform to the ethos of the marketplace, which legitimates self-interest over beneficence and makes vices out of most of medicine's traditional virtues?[3] Or should doctors stand firm in their belief that being a physician imposes specific obligations that forbid turning oneself into an entrepreneur, a businessperson, or an agent of fiscal, social, or economic policy? In this regard, Albert Jonsen, in his George Washington Gay Lectures at Harvard in 1988, looked in particular at the conflict between altruism and self-interest that is now part of the structure of modern health care. He concluded:

> History and philosophy of medicine give moral meaning to the past; moral confidence in the future can only be achieved by the scientists, administrators, and practitioners of medicine who understand its moral meaning. It is their responsibility to revise the institutions and practices created in the past without loss of moral meaning. A highly scientific medicine that reaches only a privileged minority is morally deficient. An extraordinarily competent corps of practitioners that deals only with cure and knows nothing of prevention is morally deficient. A cost-effective system of care that shuts out the dying or the elderly or the poor is morally deficient. Those responsible for the revision of medicine's past to meet its future must have confidence that they can make those revisions without sacrifice of its essential values.[4]

We do not know how the medical profession will resolve this dilemma. Many physicians still want to remain faithful to the primacy of the patient's welfare and the idea of a profession. Others see no reason why physicians should be held to a higher standard of ethical conduct than anyone else. What is most distressing is the pervasive conviction that the citadel of ethics has already fallen, that it is no longer possible to be an ethical physician, and that the only choices are capitulation, accommodation, or early retirement, with warnings to one's children not to enter the fallen city. Those who would resist feel powerless, alone, and abandoned by the profession. They justifiably complain that others cannot expect them to be sacrificial lambs trying to reverse the inimical forces arrayed against traditional medical ethics today.

To resolve the central dilemma of professional ethics, we must draw on the idea of the profession as a moral community that will use its moral power to stand against the forces eroding professional integrity, and will encourage and support those physicians within the community who have the will and the courage to adhere to traditional standards of ethical behavior.

The idea of a moral community is built into the medical profession, but it has usually remained latent or been expressed in distorted form. We wish to argue that medicine is at heart a moral community and always will be; that those who practice it are *de facto* members of a moral community, bound together by knowledge and ethical precepts; and that, as a result, physicians have collective, as well as individual, moral obligations to protect the welfare of sick persons in a world that increasingly treats medicine as a commodity, a political bauble, an investment opportunity, or a bureaucrat's power play. The profession and the public want physicians to be members of a moral community dedicated to something other than self-interest. Or are we prepared to accent instead doctors as members of a union, trade association, or political party?

To deal with these concerns, we must look at the idea of the profession as a moral community, first historically and then philosophically, and then consider the practical implications today. We will also try to determine why being a physician today makes a moral difference.

The Historical Antecedents

Let us begin with the historical antecedents. We will select five partial but flawed models of the medical community in five different eras. None of these models is completely valid. Each has some truth, and each persists in remnant form in modern collective professional consciousness.

Perhaps the first explicit model of a moral community, albeit a seriously flawed one, is contained in the opening sentences of the Hippocratic Oath.[5] Here initiates are enjoined to respect and care for their teachers as if they were their fathers, to keep the art secret, and to teach it only to their sons or the sons of other physicians. It is uncertain whether this covenant originated with the school or was added by Pythagorean thinkers.[6] A model more out of joint with contemporary sensibilities could hardly be imagined. It is secretive, sexist, paternalistic, and elitist. Commentators understandably pass over this prelude to the Oath in embarrassed silence.

But buried under this guild mentality is the nascent notion that physicians have certain responsibilities that set them apart from society. This prelude is followed by the admirable moral precepts of the body of the Oath. These precepts became the heart of the ethical commitment shared by physicians for centuries. Without giving sanction to the guild model, we can at least appreciate that it did recognize the mutual and collective responsibilities of physicians. Unfortunately, too many physicians still cling to some of the less commendable remnants of this model. They see themselves as a privileged group. They place loyalty to their professional colleagues above concern for patient welfare. They are loath to expose incompetence or to testify against colleagues in court. Clearly, while the Hippocratic model recognizes the existence of a moral community, it is morally defective because it is designed to protect the guild and not those the guild serves.

Notably absent in the Hippocratic Oath and corpus is any sense of the physician's obligations to society. Emphasis is entirely on the individual physician's duties to the individual patient. This should, of course, be primary. But no mention is made of the profession's collective obligations for the health of society, for the availability or accessibility of health care or the behavior of colleagues.[7] Paradoxically, the Stoic philosophy stressed the interrelatedness of humanity and championed benevolence toward all humans without distinction. Yet, the Stoics distrusted institutions and left medical ethics to the individual physician in the manner of the Hippocratic ethic.[8]

In the Christian era, the body of the Hippocratic Oath was preserved intact, but significantly, the offensive opening sentences were completely excluded. Presumably, this was because the church opposed secret societies. The idea of a moral community was, however, strengthened by the Christian principle of charity—unselfish love and solicitude for others, especially those who are vulnerable. This was epitomized in the idea of medicine as a vocation—a calling through which the physician worked out personal salvation by serving the needs of others.[9] The moral community for the Christian consists of the brother- and sisterhood of human beings under an all-caring Deity. The first Christian physicians were monks. Medicine thus grew up under the influence of the religious orders, often identifying with their communal charitable goals. Needless to say, not all Christian physicians, even those who were clerics, lived up to what would be expected of a moral community. Many separated their religious commitment from their professional lives, as so many physicians do today. This model, because of its religious commitment, does not have wide applicability in today's pluralistic, secular society.

The most influential model today is an attenuation of that of the physician as a member of a community of gentlemen. This model flourished in eighteenth-century England in the ethical works and persons of John and James Gregory of Edinburgh and Thomas Percival of Manchester.[10] Percival's ethics of 1803 provided all the moral precepts and even some of the words for the AMA's first code of ethics. Percival's ethic was firmly based on a clear moral philosophy. But it is the more superficial aspects of his gentlemanly model that have shaped Anglo-American medical ethics. In Percival, as in the AMA code, much space is given to the obligations physicians owe to each other, especially with respect to consultations. As a member of a gentleman's club, the doctor was held to the rules of interpersonal etiquette, to provide care for the poor and to be solicitous and compassionate to the sick.

The gentleman doctor was part of a community of privilege to be sure. But to a greater degree than in previous eras, he (and sometimes she) had responsibility for socially important problems like the health of workers, the design of hospitals for the insane, and forensic medicine. This sense of the wider obligation of the medical community was epitomized in the words of Benjamin Rush: "they entertain very limited views of medicine who suppose its object and duties are confined exclusively to the knowledge and cure of diseases. Our science was intended to render other services to society."[11]

Remnants of this gentlemanly model of the medical community persist among older physicians today. While this model had certain virtues, it is not sufficient for our times. It has too much of the aura of privilege and condescension to suit today's democratic, antielitist, and egalitarian social mores. But granting its deficiencies, the eighteenth-century model had certain virtues that could properly qualify it as a moral community.

Medicine as a Moral Community

Many factors in recent years have converged to weaken the eighteenth-century idea of medicine as a community. Specialization has divided the body of knowledge formerly held in common into dozens of pieces; medical ethics itself has focused on decision-making by individual physicians and has given little attention to their collective obligations; moral pluralism divides physicians as it does everyone else. As a result, the Hippocratic ethic itself is no longer a unifying factor. Many physicians now reject one or another of its precepts—for example, the proscriptions against abortion and euthanasia. We can hardly say what constitutes the ethics of medicine today. To this we must add legitimation of the profit motive, the transformation of the physician into a variety of roles—businessperson, scientist, proletarian, corporate executive. Each of these new roles draws the physician into a separate community foreign to medicine and further weakens the moral identification with its traditional ethic. This separation is inimical to the notion of the healing community.

Moreover, whatever sense of community there may be in medicine is sometimes expressed in a seriously distorted way. One thinks of the defensive and retaliatory stance of the profession to some of the admittedly hostile intrusions of law, government, consumer groups, and the like. Here the motive is not protection of the patient against policies and practices deleterious to patient care. Rather, it is a tit-for-tat, sometimes vindictive reaction expressed in a refusal to provide care for the needy, for the unsavory patient, or even for lawyers or their families. This is a return to the guild mentality with a vengeance. In a similar way, when physicians strike, as they have done in some parts of the world, their community is the community of a union, not of a profession, of self-interest, not of activism.

This deterioration of the idea of medicine as a moral community has had a serious impact on the profession and society. There is no collective professional voice speaking for the patient, resisting practices that undermine ethics or endanger patient care. Indeed, we are hard put to define the common content of medical ethics. Physicians who resist are morally abandoned to defend themselves, without encouragement or support from their profession. Only the most courageous raise their voices, and at great risk of retribution even from their professional colleagues. The enormous moral power that resides in the community of medicine is left unused.

The Philosophical Foundation of the Moral Community

Let us step back from these realities for a moment and see why medicine cannot escape being a moral community. Three things about medicine as a human activity make it a moral enterprise that imposes collective responsibilities of great moment on its practitioners: (1) the nature of illness, (2) the nonproprietary nature of medical knowledge, and (3) the nature and circumstances of a professional oath.

First is the nature of illness itself, because it is illness, as a universal human phenomenon, that makes medicine a special kind of human activity. The sick person is in a uniquely dependent, anxious, vulnerable, and exploitable state. Sick persons must bare their weaknesses, compromise their dignity, and reveal intimacies of body and mind. The predicament of illness forces them to trust the physician in a relationship that they would prefer not to enter and in which they are relatively powerless. Moreover, when the physician invites the patient's trust, he or she offers to put professional knowledge at the service of the patient. Illness is an assault upon the whole person. The existence of a genuine medical need constitutes a moral claim on those equipped to help.[12] This claim forges a common bond between those who need help and those who profess to help.

Second, the physician's knowledge is not proprietary. It is acquired through the privilege of a medical education. Society sanctions certain invasions of privacy such as dissecting and performing autopsies on human bodies, participating in the care of the sick, or experimenting with human subjects. These actions would be illegal in circumstances other than medical education. The student is permitted free access to all of the world's medical knowledge, much of it gained by observation and experimentation on generations of sick persons. Doctors, through licensing, credentialing, and certification, are promised a monopoly by society over the usual medical knowledge. All of this, and even financial subsidization of medical education, are permitted for one purpose—to ensure that society has an uninterrupted supply of trained medical personnel.

The physician's knowledge therefore is not private property. Nor is it intended primarily for personal gain, prestige, or power. Rather, the profession holds medical knowledge in trust for the good of the sick. By accepting the privilege of a medical education, those who enter medicine become parties to a covenant with society— one that cannot be dissolved unilaterally. Medical students, from their first day, enter a community bound by a moral covenant. They accept the privileges of medical education in return for the responsibility of stewardship of medical knowledge.

Moreover, this covenant is acknowledged publicly when the physician takes an oath at graduation. The oath—not the degree—symbolizes the graduate's formal entry into the profession. The oath—whichever one is taken—is a public promise— a "profession"—that the new physician understands the gravity of his or her calling, promises to be competent, and promises to use that competence in the interests of the sick. Some effacement of self-interest is thus intrinsic to every medical oath. That is what makes medicine truly a profession.[13]

These three things—the nature of illness, the nonproprietary character of medical knowledge, and the oath of fidelity to the patient's interests—generate a strong moral bond and a collective responsibility. To place self-interest ahead of the interest of the patient thus is to abnegate the very essence of what it is to be a physician. The physician is no more free to flee from danger in the performance of his or her duties than the fireman, the policeman, or the soldier. The physician cannot shirk those duties by shrugging them off on willing colleagues or remain indifferent to those who deny their obligations.

Two divergent ethical conceptions of medicine therefore oppose each other today. One favors individualism, self-interest, isolation from one's fellows, and accommodation to whatever society or patients demand. The other recognizes that the physician has ethical obligations that transcend self-interests, exigency, and even social, political, and economic forces. If they are in fact members of a moral community, doctors must be faithful to the moral binding forces in that community. They must concentrate on what it is to be a good physician and what kind of person that physician should be.

If physicians are truly members of a moral community, the public can expect that they will not take advantage of the patient's vulnerability; that they will not use patients as means to their own ends—profit, prestige, power; that they can be trusted to act in the patient's best interests even if it may cost time, effort, or money or expose them to risk. These are not things we normally expect of a business, where by contrast the competitor's vulnerability is something to be exploited, where personal self-interest, profit, and market dominance are sometimes primary goals, and indeed are the very incentives that drive the entrepreneur.

If physicians are faithful to the moral obligations they share as a community, then it is clear that some of the role transformations being forced upon physicians today ought to be rejected. Health professionals cannot become primarily business-persons, entrepreneurs, bureaucrats, proletarians, or corporate employees. Health and health care cannot become commodities whose price, availability, accessibility, and distribution are determined by market forces. Nor can health care be primarily an industry, an opportunity for investment, or an instrument of social policy. The metaphors of business and industry signal a downward drift in moral expectations. They are not the metaphors of a moral community. Physicians have a collective responsibility to resist and reveal this moral down drift.

This downward drift is a great danger to the profession and to the public. It discourages the most sensitive and responsible members of the profession. We can understand why physicians are reluctant to imperil their families, their careers, and their livelihoods. But it is a moral judgment upon all of them if they allow their most ethical colleagues to go unsupported.

What Is the "Good Physician" to Do?

How shall we respond when conscientious physicians ask, "What is a good person to do?" Physicians are neither saints nor heroes. We cannot expect individuals to solve all the problems associated with practicing medicine in today's money culture and morally chaotic times. But there is still much we can do—as individuals and collectively as a community supporting this profession.

First, let us recognize that part of physicians' moral desuetude lies within the body of healers—not simply with lawyers, government bureaucrats, legislators, or insurance companies. As individuals they must still answer to their own consciences. They must form their consciences in recognition of the fact that they are engaged in an activity that is essentially different from commerce, trade, or craft. They are committed, by the nature of what is required to care for a sick person, to a level of beneficence that goes beyond the minimalistic requirements of law, which merely forbids harming others. No fiscal exigency, no political, social, or technological change, can extirpate the roots of a doctor's moral obligation.

The physician—and the nurse and other health professionals as well—are at the moral center of health care. They are society's delegated advocates for the sick. Ultimately, they are the instruments through which health policies are implemented. They are the final common pathway through which all that happens to the patients must go. They have enormous moral power if they choose to exercise it. No one can make health professionals do what is thought to be harmful to patients. As long as the reasons for resistance encompass the good of the sick, doctors can prevail against unethical practices and policies and win public support for their resistance. Unfortunately, their collective protestations as professional societies are often so patently self-serving that they lose all moral credibility.

There is still much that doctors can do as individuals. They can restrain self-interest when the good of the patient requires it. They can refuse those financial incentives that seduce others into dubious practices. They can examine fees or their overeager use of fee-producing techniques. They can do more to care for the poor and those on the margins of society. Doctors can resist the distorted notion of justice that says that it's just too bad if you happen to be a member of one of the less fortunate segments of society. Resisting, physicians might refuse to indulge in economic transfer, the "yellow professionalism"[14] of misleading advertising, or the conflict of interest in referring patients to the laboratory, MRI unit, or dialysis unit that they may own. These are things we expect of the virtuous physician, as we shall see later in this work.

Physicians need to be better schooled in medical ethics because ultimately it is the only discipline that places moral restraint on self-interest. Ethics aims to make us more critical of what we are doing—to bring us back daily to thinking about what it is to be a good doctor. What does it mean to be a professional? Is the downward moral drift afflicting me as an individual? Are individual physicians becoming the kinds of persons and doctors that I could not in good conscience defend? When am I morally compelled to disobey a policy or law that goes against the welfare of the sick person?

If we fail to be critical about morality, we lose our capacity to recognize moral evil. Today medicine, in practice and academia, is making a series of Faustian moral compacts with business, government, and even science. Fiscal survival and exigency are the usual moral justifications, although reasons of greater productivity and faster service are often advanced. As in all Faustian compacts, Mephistopheles will sooner or later show up to claim his part of the bargain—to claim many professional souls. The distance between self-interest and greed, between Machiavelli and Mephistopheles, is short.

It is tragic that the good physician, the one with the right motivations, is so often left to resist the current downward moral drift left alone. This is a moral indictment of the whole profession. Each physician has made an individual act of "pro-fession," a promise of disinterested service. But he or she has also made a collective promise to serve the sick. The profession as a whole has an obligation to advocate the welfare of the sick. Just as each individual health care provider is the advocate for his or her own patients, the profession should raise its voice in accord with one ordering principle—the primacy of the patient's well-being. To be sure, as a profession, physicians have argued strenuously against certain governmental and local policies inimical to patient care. But they have often done so out of self-interest—because these suggested policies and laws violate their own prerogatives. Such arguments will be effective only if they can show how a policy erodes the covenant with the sick person. When a health care professional says, "Can I help you?," that caregiver raises the expectation that he or she will help. The professional is morally obliged to meet that expectation.

The medical profession had enormous power for moral good. We do not think it has exercised this power as fully or effectively as it might in these days of tremendous moral challenge. If doctors as a healing community really want to recapture a sense of moral integrity, the most important thing they can do is to resist and to refuse to do anything that violates the promise to act in the patient's interests. There are times when there is a moral obligation to disobey. Doctors who are older and in positions of influence bear a greater responsibility to resist than those who are younger and do not have the freedom and independence, professionally or financially, that their seniors enjoy.

Were physicians to take moral leadership, the medical profession could be a model and an inspiration for the others. Law is in the same, or worse, moral confusion and, as recent events so sensationally show, so is the ministry—at least in its electronic incarnations. We must not miss the fact that medicine has taken the lead among the professions in the current renaissance of concern for ethics. Colleagues in the other professions are, as a consequence, also beginning to stir.

Today's revolution in medical ethics is profound in its social significance. It is more significant than anything that has happened in the 2500-year history of medicine and medical ethics. We are in the midst of a genuine dismantling of a noble and ancient edifice.

Nonetheless, it is still possible to be an ethical physician in an ethical profession; indeed, unless doctors wish to lose their moral integrity, they must be so. To make this possible, they must for the first time in medical history establish themselves as a true moral community, as a group of persons dedicated to something other than their own self-interest, as a group that recognizes its responsibility to support the ethical members of its company, to repel or reject those who are not faithful to the ethical bonds that unite the community, and to advocate the cause of the sick, even when society and politics militate against it. These duties flow not only from the characteristics of the healing community described in the previous section, but also from the qualities of professional commitment.

The medical profession today is afflicted by a siege mentality. Its members are acting like the occupants of a citadel about to fall into the hands of hostile forces. Like the occupants of a besieged city, they are divided, dispirited, and tempted to defect. Worst of all, physicians are becoming convinced that the traditional sources of the profession's credibility, its moral commitments, have no survival value in today's competitive climate. Only a fool, many would say, would rely on moral weaponry in today's morally unscrupulous environment.

This dolorous scenario is without moral justification, and it is self-defeating. It is precisely because health professionals have not been entirely faithful to their collective moral obligations that they are in danger of being overwhelmed. As we have taken pains to elaborate, physicians are *de facto* members of a moral community of healers. Were they to use the moral power they possess, they could neutralize and reverse the forces eroding the profession.

But to do so, they must take the high moral ground. The profession must admit its own errors, correct them, and take leadership on the only defensible ground, which is not its own self-interest but the interests of those who health care providers profess to serve. Physicians must choose between two worlds: one governed by the virtues and rules of ethics and concern for the patient, the other by the rules of politics, economics, and self-interest.

Does It Make a Moral Difference to Be a Physician?

There are two very disturbing questions today in the medical profession. One is: What difference does it make to be a physician? The second is: What difference does it make to be a virtuous physician? Both questions are pertinent to the idea of a moral community that we have just been discussing.

Corollaries of the first of the questions are: Why should physicians be expected to adhere to a system of ethics that requires more of them than of other persons in our society? Why should physicians try to suppress self-interest, at great cost to their own welfare and that of their families, when other professionals pursue self-interest with singular determination? We have addressed these questions philosophically in earlier works.[15] There we argued that the nature of **the healing relationship** is itself the foundation for the special obligations of physicians as physicians. These obligations, we hold, are binding on all physicians.

Here we turn to the second question: What difference does it make to be a physician? This question asks whether anything is required beyond what is derivable for all other human beings. This is a timely question, since many physicians are unclear about their identity and behavior, and about how to reconcile profession and virtues in a secular, pluralistic society.

It is a dictum that "ought implies can," that is, that we cannot require a particular obligation in practice, however justifiable theoretically, if the agent cannot, for some good reason, perform it. We argue that physicians are indeed required to observe particular obligations in practice, irrespective of what the mores of our society may be, and that in addition, it is possible—though difficult—to fulfill those obligations even in the morally vexed state of society today. The challenge goes to the heart of what it is to *be* a physician. Much of the disaffection, distress, and cynicism that beset physicians relates to their confusion and uncertainty about the answers to the two questions we pose. Yet how we answer these questions largely determines the moral quality of the medical enterprise as a profession, the satisfaction individuals derive from it, and the degree of dedication society can expect from them to the interests of the sick rather than their own.

The Moral Climate of Medical Practice

Before we address each question separately, let us sketch the reasons for the urgency of these questions today.

In the past, some physicians questioned the constraints on their behavior imposed by traditional medical moralists. But they were a minority, and there was little social or ethical sanction for any significant departure from traditional medical morality. To be sure, the actual performance of physicians has not always conformed to the ideal. The world's literature is filled with satirical portrayals of our profession's moral failings. But if in the past there were doubts about the doctor's actual ethical behavior, there was little doubt about what his or her behavior *ought* to be.

What is so different today is that policymakers, patients, ethicists, and physicians themselves, each for their own reasons, are urging conceptions of what physicians ought to be that are radically at variance with traditional ethics. Policymakers want physicians to be gatekeepers of society's resources and instruments of the bureaucratic apparatus; patients want absolute autonomy and see health professionals increasingly as instruments of their wishes; ethicists want to substitute a contractual for a fiduciary model of the physician–patient relationship;[16] administrators of managed-care systems want doctors to be entrepreneurs, competitors, and instruments of profit. Physicians' capabilities are demeaned, on the one hand, as too technological, while on the other they are endowed with such magical powers that they are held liable for the fallibilities of nature itself. Doctors are sued for doing too much and for doing too little. Fiscal incentives and disincentives are used to modify professional behavior, and then physicians are chastised for responding.

In the face of such a confusion of voices, is it surprising that physicians ask, why should we practice effacement of self-interest when everyone else is pursuing self-interest? How can we advocate the interests of the patient when there are so many intrusions into that relationship? To make matters worse, we must confront these questions without the moral moorings that provided some security in the past. Moral pluralism, moral neutrality, or amoralism are the order of the day. The Hippocratic Oath and ethos have been reshaped to fit our society's changing mores.[17] Every one of its precepts is challenged—even the primacy of beneficence.[18] Most of the complex ethical challenges they face were not imaginable until a few decades ago. Finally, the most fundamental human life issues have been detached from their religious foundations, so that human conception, living, and dying are no longer sacred precincts but simply another opportunity for technological prestidigitation.

Are physicians and other health professionals not justified, then, in their confusion? Who can blame them for being depressed, besieged, cynical, hostile, and at times even vindictive? For some, the only alternatives seem to be early retirement, compromise with actions that make them morally uncomfortable, or comfortable accommodation. Some say that this is the way it ought to be. For others, this is a new world and they welcome it. They might say: "The Federal Trade Commission says we are a business; let us take advantage of it while it lasts. We are what society makes us. Everything else is a business, and so is medicine. We owe nothing to patients except competence. We need not extend ourselves, since they will sue us no matter what we do. Survival is the name of the game."

This is a sample of the disquieting attitudes one hears expressed recurrently about, and by, physicians. Even Dr. Pangloss' proverbial optimism might be dampened by prospects of rescuing the remnants of moral integrity in such an unpromising climate.[19] Yet this is precisely what must and can be done. We have seen what the exercise of moral power can accomplish in Eastern Europe in circumstances far more burdensome than those the medical profession faces. Have physicians lost all moral convictions? Can the profession justify the loss of moral convictions in a matter of such importance to human well-being?

Why Must Physicians Be Subject to Moral Constraints?

Let us turn then to our first question. Why are medicine and the health professions called to a certain standard of moral behavior, even if the society around them permits or even encourages less constraining moral attitudes? We will concentrate on the imperative most central to being a profession and indispensable for medical morality—**effacement of self-interest**. It is precisely at this point that the moral quality of medicine's whole enterprise is most clearly revealed. Many physicians feel they must protect self-interest or they cannot survive in today's hostile practice environment. Why should physicians and other health professions suppress self-interest?

Reference to professional codes is insufficient. Codes are expressions of moral beliefs, but they are not self-justifying. They must be based on something more fundamental, on a philosophy of medicine, particularly on the central distinguishing moral features of medical activity, that is, the healing relationship between one who is ill and one who professes to help and heal. It is in doubts about the healing relationship that doubts about traditional medical ethics have their origin. The healing relationship is the moral fulcrum, the archimedean point at which the balance between self-interest and self-effacement must be struck.

Let us cite five features that characterize the specific human relationship medicine entails. These are what provides medicine its moral imperatives.[20] Taken together, these imperatives constitute an "internal morality" of medicine—something built into the nature of medicine as a particular kind of human activity. They are (1) the inequality of the medical relationship, (2) the fiduciary nature of the relationship, (3) the moral nature of medical decisions, (4) the nature of medical knowledge, and (5) the ineradicable moral complicity of the physician in whatever happens to the patient.

1. Vulnerability and inequality. A central phenomenon of illness is the vulnerability of the sick person and the consequent inequality it introduces into the medical relationship. Even the most self-sufficient person becomes anxious, fearful, and dependent when illness occurs. Patients experience loss of freedom—to pursue life's goals, to make their own decisions, and to heal themselves without access to specialized knowledge and skill. Pursuit of relief, cure, and return to health become central preoccupations. In this state, the sick person is forced to consult another person who professes to hold the needed knowledge and skill and who, therefore, has power over the ill person.

These facts impose a condition of existential inequality on the medical relationship paralleled by few other situations in democratic societies. Taken together, they engender a state of unusual vulnerability. This inescapable vulnerability imposes *de facto* moral obligations on the physician. In a relationship of such inequality, the weight of obligations is on the one with the power. This is very different from the ethos of business, where vulnerability is an opportunity to exploit one's competitor. The physician instead has the obligation to protect the vulnerability of the patient against exploitation.

2. Fiduciary nature of the relationship. In this condition of vulnerability, patients are forced to trust physicians. They may scrutinize credentials, reputations, and performance, but at some point they must trust one member of the profession—the one they have finally chosen. Trust is ineradicable, despite the fact that some ethicists today would do away with it by substituting the contract model.[21] But what contract can anticipate all the decisions we make even in a supposedly simple case? Patients must, sooner or later, expose and reveal themselves to be healed and helped—expose their bodies, their minds, and at times even their souls and failings. Moreover, physicians invite their trust—as individuals, when they ask, "How can I help you?", and as a profession, when they take a public oath at commencement. That oath is a public promise that they belong to a special kind of community, one dedicated to something other than self-interest, that they possess knowledge and will use it for the benefit of those who need it.

3. The nature of medical decisions. The third thing that makes the medical relationship a moral enterprise is the fact the most serious medical decisions combine technical and moral components. The physician must be scientifically correct in making a diagnosis, prognosis, and choice of therapy but, at the same time, his or her recommendation must be for the patient's good. The latter includes more than the patient's medical good.[22] The patient's moral right to self-determination must be respected. The physician must assess the moral status of the recommendation. The physician must also decide whether his or her own moral beliefs are consistent with what the patient requests. There are moral issues, of course, in all human relationships, but because of the special vulnerability and exploitability of the sick person and the fiduciary relationships, these moral issues assume overriding importance in medical relationships. The good of the patient is the end and purpose of that relationship. But this is as much a moral as a technical good. To see the relationship between the technical and moral aspects of medical decisions, and to place them in the right relationship to each other, is an inescapable moral obligation and the test of a true physician.

4. The characteristics of medical knowledge. Medical knowledge has certain characteristics that generate obligations in those who possess it. For one thing, it is practical knowledge, knowledge intended for a specific purpose—the care of the sick. It is not knowledge acquired *primarily* for its own sake. In addition, medical knowledge is obtained only through the socially sanctioned privilege of a medical education. Society permits the invasions of the privacy of sick persons that medical education demands. Students are allowed to dissect human bodies, see autopsies, engage in experimentation, practice their skills, and gain experience in clinical care. These privileges cannot be bought for a price, like other commodities. No tuition could generate a right to the invasions of privacy required in medical education. Moreover, financial subsidization is provided by society to ensure an uninterrupted supply of medical personnel, not to provide students with a means of future livelihood.

We must not forget that physicians are granted a monopoly over medical knowledge. Physicians still enjoy wide discretionary latitude in the use of medical knowledge. They are allowed freedom to accredit educational programs and set standards of practice, to admit to and eject physicians from the medical community. This creates in the profession a reciprocal collective responsibility to ensure that medical knowledge is available, accessible, and accurate, and that it is used within definite ethical constraints. The physician's knowledge can never be his or her private property because medical knowledge is entrusted to the profession for the care of the sick. Physicians are its stewards, not its exploiters. As stewards, they are obliged to preserve, validate, teach, and extend medical knowledge and see that it is available and accessible to those for whom it is acquired in the first place. Medical knowledge can never be a commodity since, unlike commodities, it is produced not for its exchange value but because it is needed by sick human beings.

5. Moral complicity. The physician, by virtue of the covenant and the way medicine is practiced, is the final common pathway for whatever happens to a patient. No order can be carried out, no policy observed, and no regulation imposed without the physician's assent. It is the physician who writes the orders that other health professionals carry out. He or she is inescapably the final safeguard of the patient's well-being. The physician is therefore *de facto* a moral accomplice in whatever is done for good or ill to patients. The physician cannot be a double agent; he or she serves primarily the patient or primarily the self, the hospital, the economic or fiscal policy, or the law. This ultimate responsibility is not transferable to others even in these days of team care, ethics communities, and court decisions. Without the cooperation of physicians, the Nazi homicides would not have been possible.[23] Nor would the exploitation of the sick for profit.

These five characteristics of **the healing relationship** constitute the moral ground for the answer to the first question: Why must physicians be held to higher standards of effacement of self-interest than others in our society? Analogous phenomena characterize the nurse–patient, the minister–parishioner, and even the lawyer–client relationship. Each relationship implies a distinctive set of moral imperatives that shape their internal moralities and defines the moral nature of their enterprises. The nature of medical activity is such that self-interest, however strong and universal, must to a degree be suppressed in the interest of sick persons. The nature of the activity of medicine precludes the Hobbesian stance of self-interest as the primary motive for human conduct.

Is It Possible to Be an Ethical Physician Today?

What about the second question? Even if these arguments are granted, is it possible to be faithful to the moral requirements of the healing relationship and to survive in a world in which the pursuit of self-interest is dominant and widely legitimated? Wasn't Machiavelli right—the virtuous person is not likely to survive when everyone else is being nonvirtuous? How about Hobbes—"glory and profit" are the *only* human motives? Recall that Bernard Mandeville, a fellow physician, insisted that society could not thrive without cultivating the vices because satisfying them was the engine that fueled the economy.[24]

We think these antivirtue philosophers are wrong. Physicians *can* be ethical.

However, it will probably be difficult for all but the most courageous among them, unless they recognize the five morality-demanding characteristics of medicine as a certain kind of human activity. In addition, they must cultivate an old and neglected ideal: the ideal of a moral community, the idea of physicians and other health professionals bound, by their common commitment to care for the sick, to a set of shared and collective obligations. As we have noted, a moral community is one that effaces its group interests before the higher interests that give it its definitive character.

Historically, we have been accustomed to think only in terms of the obligations of individual physicians to individual patients. Certainly, the person of character is still the indispensable unit of a morally good society. Yet, given today's practice milieu, individual physicians cannot be expected to meet their ethical obligations singlehandedly. Even the virtuous physician will need a virtuous community to provide support. The idea of collective obligations, except to advance self-interest, is foreign to our usual conceptions of professional ethics.

We do not wish to ignore the fact that in many ways the profession, through its national, state, or local societies and hospital staffs, has manifested awareness of the idea of a moral community. We can cite, as a few examples, affirmation of the moral obligation to treat patients with HIV infection; the conscientious fulfillment of peer review responsibilities; the updating of ethical codes and guidelines; the stance of the profession with respect to preventive medicine, notably with respect to smoking, fatty diets, exercise, use of drugs, alcohol, safe driving, seat belts, boxing injuries, and care for the poor and the homeless; establishing standards of medical education; and the recent American College of Physicians' and American Medical Association's recognition of the problems of accessibility of health care.[25]

These are all commendable evidence of collective professional responsibility. But they do not address the more sensitive issue of professional self-interest and the advocacy role the professional should play in the conflict between an ethic based in the marketplace and one based in the moral nature of the medical relationship. Without in any way depreciating what is being done by many conscientious individual physicians and their organizations, the full spectrum of our obligations as a moral community are yet to be fulfilled. Medicine has yet to use the tremendous moral power it possesses for good. To do so, it must act collectively in certain ways.[26]

Physicians should begin by examining themselves and admitting that not all of the fault for the parlous state of medical care today lies outside the profession. To be sure, the *bêtes noires* are not imaginary—the malpractice crisis, inimical public and regulative policies, insurance carrier venality, corporations ducking responsibility for health care, the ethos of the marketplace replete with its advertising, competition, "bottom-line" administrators, for-profit hospitals, meaningless paperwork, and so on. The list is long and distressing. The tendency to blame current moral desuetude on the "climate" of medical practice is understandable and in part justifiable. But we must also realize that self-righteous complaints are self-serving. They seriously compromise moral integrity. Integrity can be restored by taking the moral high ground, by acting not on the basis of what external forces do to the profession, but on what they do to those who are served.

Some of the wounds inflicted on the body of the profession are self-generated. Some physicians have refused to see Medicare and Medicaid patients, to treat HIV infection, to go to the emergency room, or to do any *pro bono* work. Some physicians have defrauded their patients, the Medicare/Medicaid system, or third-party payers. Some physicians charge unconscionable fees, are unavailable when needed, and are overly protective of their colleagues in the face of incompetence or venality. We emphasize *some* physicians. The majority have not done these things. But we must acknowledge that the current climate of antipathy is not the result of a massive conspiracy against the profession. If there is a moral community, physicians are all touched by the virtues and vices of confreres. They must feel demeaned by the latter and act to repudiate them. They must also admit moral aberrations. This experience alone leads us to argue throughout the book that emphasis on the virtues is insufficient for a moral outcome.

One should take a stand against the evils inside and outside of medicine on one ground only—the damage and danger they pose for the sick. Every one of the things that disturb conscientious physicians—in their colleagues' behavior or in today's social milieu—can be effectively opposed if physicians are faithful to the central aim of medicine, which is the care and cure of the sick. Were they to take this position, they would have public sentiment with them. Physicians must demonstrate that their first concern is not their own privileges, prerogatives, or income, but the welfare of those they have a covenant to serve. There is enormous moral power in this position.

Advocacy of the sick will be an empty gesture, or interpreted as another public relations gimmick, if it is not accompanied by actions. There are a variety of efforts that organized medicine—or new associations of physicians—can undertake to make the profession's advocacy role authentic and effective.

Physicians should collect the data needed to convince the public and legislators that the free market, commercialization, and monetarization of medicine are unjust and damaging to the welfare of the sick. Anecdotal accounts are not sufficient to make the case, impressive as they may be. If there is clear evidence that a given policy is injurious to patients, physicians must resist and even refuse to carry it out. No policy can make all of America's physicians do what they think is morally wrong. To comply is to be an accomplice in violation of the covenant with the sick patient.

The profession should resist the uncritical acceptance of the idea that rationing of health care is necessary in America. Even a superficial comparison between the magnitude of health expenditures and the ways we spend billions of dollars in discretionary income should convince us that needed medical care need not be withheld. Before physicians talk about rationing, they can take steps to reduce the waste of resources in unnecessary and duplicated workups, procedures, operations, and medications. They can fight to reduce the administrative overhead (15–30% in the opinion of some economists) imposed on health care expenditures by "managed" health care systems, with their administrative bureaucracies, advertising and marketing budgets, and the whole cumbersome and expensive paper chase that buries both the physician and the patient.[27]

The profession must initiate and cooperate with efforts to eliminate excessive fees by adopting a fee schedule and a relative value-scale system of compensation. Investment in health care facilities and other forms of conflict of interest are ethically unacceptable. Physicians, by virtue of their heavy responsibilities, are entitled to just compensation. But they must not regard themselves as entrepreneurs with a monopoly and a franchise to exploit medical knowledge. Physicians should heed the plea of the editor of the *Journal of the American Medical Association* and others for a return to the tradition of *pro bono* work for the poor as part of the responsibility of every physician.[28]

What America, the sick among us, and the health care system need desperately is moral leadership and medical statesmanship. That leadership cannot be effected by individual physicians acting alone. But acting as a moral community, the profession has enormous power to resist the forces it finds so inimical to the well-being of its patients and its own well-being through that power. It can influence the public, government, and industry to reevaluate their values and to appreciate that the fulfillment of each person's potential is impossible without health and medical care for all citizens.

Medicine cannot, and should not, undertake all of this alone. It can join with other health professional, concerned people, and legislators. We do not need more reports from commissions, panels, and committees on how to solve the health care "crisis" by still another prescription for tinkering with the mechanisms. The answer is clear: America can have health quality care for all if we order our priorities as a nation; if health professionals dedicate themselves to the care of the sick as their primary obligation, and not to their own self-interest; and if our health professions together take leadership in persuading Americans to be a caring, rather than a mean-spirited and acquisitive, society, unwilling to make any sacrifice for the vulnerable among us.

The idea of medicine as a moral community is very old. Yet, for the greater part of our history, this idea has been only latent or expressed in a nascent form. It is present in distorted form in the opening paragraphs of the Hippocratic Oath. Here new physicians are enjoined to treat their teachers as fathers, their sons as brothers, and to teach the art only to their own sons or those of their teachers. The spirit of this covenant is so frankly sexist, paternalistic, and elitist that it offends our democratic sensibilities—as it should. But it does carry the idea of a community bound together by a common commitment—namely, the substance of the oath that follows it. Those ideals have given us a common identity for a long time.

Should health care reshape its ethos to conform to the marketplace, as Engelhardt counsels,[29] or should it stand firm in the belief that medicine imposes specific obligations that, by the nature of what the physician does and is, preclude being primarily a business person, entrepreneur or agent of social or fiscal policy?

Medicine has the opportunity to provide society with evidence of at least one group that acts from something more than self-interest. To do so, the profession must respond in the affirmative to the two questions with which we opened this section: Yes, more is demanded of physicians than others in society. Yes, they can be ethical in today's practice climate. To act in this way is to adopt the virtues, some of which we examine in this work. But how should the project of reconstituting the profession of medicine proceed today?

Where to Turn?

Robert Veatch has long recognized that the lay–professional relationship, formerly on a somewhat solid ethical footing, must now be reanalyzed. In part this is due to the rapid changes in the balance of power in that relationship, especially with the now dominant emphasis on the principle of patient autonomy. But in part, too, the change is due to the way in which the professions once regulated themselves, and are now highly regulated by external forces, forces such as the government, third-party payers, economic factors, and the like. The latter are the focus of Veatch's work, particularly his views of justice and the social contract. He notes:

> To build an ethic for the lay–professional relationship, we must go back to the basic principles of the first or social contract. . . . In the professional ethics discussed and rejected [earlier in the book], the professions themselves generated or at least articulated the ethical principles or norms for the professional role. They sometimes went so far as to define the moral requirements for the lay person for the professional relation as well.[30]

This turn to the social contract grounds Veatch's argument that the Hippocratic ethic is dead.

In this chapter we have suggested a different approach for reconstituting an ethic for medicine. A return to the social contract is only part of the picture. Indeed, we disagree with one of Veatch's central contentions: that the medical community has no right to develop its own professional standards, and that a key feature of remapping a new social contract is that only society has that right. In later chapters, we will give reasons why medical ethics must maintain a certain distance from society's mores. We will argue that the integrity of medical ethics has an internal validity. Medicine indeed has an obligation to attend to and balance its social responsibilities, but not at the expense of a social redefinition of its ethics that might vitiate many moral aims of medical relationships.

We deem it essential to emphasize the virtuous requirements of the physician in a changing and pluralistic moral climate. To be sure, some of the more formal expectations, rules, guidelines, principles, and the like acquire their moral force within the context of human relationships. The social contract is precisely a theory of social obligations. However, the very nature of the social contract and its implementation depends upon the moral character of the participants.[31] This entails a role for virtue ethics no matter what model of the physician–patient relationship we adopt. This point, then, leads us to examine the ends of medicine and the virtues of the discipline itself, for in relationship to those ends, the virtues acquire their justification and employment.

Notes

1. Michael Oakeshott, *"Rationalism in Politics" and Other Essays* (Indianapolis: Liberty Press, 1991), p. 295.

2. Alasdair MacIntyre, *Three Rival Versions of Moral Enquiry: Encyclopedia, Geneology, and Tradition* (Notre Dame, IN: University of Notre Dame Press, 1990), p. 139.

3. H. T. Engelhardt, Jr., and M. A. Rie, "Morality for the Medical-Industrial Complex: A Code of Ethics for the Mass Marketing of Health Care," *New England Journal of Medicine* 319 (October 20, 1989): 1086–1089.

4. Albert Jonsen, *The New Medicine and the Old Ethics* (Cambridge, MA.: Harvard University Press, 1990).

5. "To hold my teacher in this art equal to my own parents; to make him partner in my livelihood; when he is in need of money to share mine with him; to consider his family as my own brothers; and to teach them this art, if they want to learn it, without fee or indenture; to impart precept, oral instruction, and all other instruction to my own sons, the sons of my teacher, and to indentured pupils who have taken the physician's oath, but to nobody else"—Hippocrates, *Oath*, in *Hippocrates I*, Loeb Classic Library, trans. W. H. S. Jones (Cambridge, MA: Harvard University Press, 1962), p. 299.

6. Ludwig Edelstein, *Ancient Medicine: Selected Papers of Ludwig Edelstein*, ed. O. Temkin and C. L. Temkin (Baltimore, MD: Johns Hopkins University Press, 1967), pp. 40–57; W. H. S. Jones, *The Doctor's Oath: An Essay in the History of Medicine* (Cambridge: Cambridge University Press, 1924), pp. 42–45; P. Carrick, *Medical Ethics in Antiquity: Philosophical Perspectives on Abortion* (Dordrecht, Holland: Kluwer, 1985), pp. 76–77.

7. Edmund D. Pellegrino, "Toward an Expanded Medical Ethics: The Hippocratic Ethics Revisited," *In Search of the Modern Hippocrates*, ed. R. Bulger (Iowa City: University of Iowa Press, 1987), pp. 45–64.

8. Giovanni Reale, *The Systems of the Hellenic Age: A History of Ancient Philosophy*, ed. and trans. John Catan (Buffalo: State University of New York Press, 1985), pp. 282–283.

9. Edmund D. Pellegrino, "Towards a Reconstruction of Medical Morality: The Primacy of the Act of Profession and the Fact of Illness," *Journal of Medicine and Philosophy* 4(1) (March 1979):32–56.

10. Thomas Percival, *Medical Ethics* (Birmingham: Classics of Medicine Library, 1985).

11. Benjamin Rush, *The Selected Writings of Benjamin Rush* Ed. Dagobert D. Runes (New York: Philosophical Library, 1947).

12. Edmund D. Pellegrino and David C. Thomasma, *A Philosophical Basis of Medical Practice* (New York: Oxford University Press, 1981).

13. Edmund D. Pellegrino and Alice A. Pellegrino, "Humanism and Ethics in Roman Medicine: Translation and Commentary on a Text of Scribonius Largus," *Literature and Medicine* 7 (1988):22–38.

14. J. M. Reade and R. M. Ratzan, "Yellow Journalism: Advertising by Physicians in the Yellow Pages," *New England Journal of Medicine* 316(21) (May, 21 1987):1315–1319.

15. Edmund D. Pellegrino and David C. Thomasma, *A Philosophical Basis of Medical Practice* (New York: Oxford University Press, 1981) and *For the Patient's Good: Toward the Restoration of Beneficence in Health Care* (New York: Oxford University Press, 1988).

16. See Robert Veatch, "Is Trust of Professionals a Coherent Concept?", *Ethics, Trust, and the Professions: Philosophical and Cultural Aspects* ed. Edmund D. Pellegrino, Robert M. Veatch, and John P. Langan (Washington, DC: Georgetown University Press, 1991), pp. 159–176; Allen Buchanan, "The Physician's Knowledge and the Patient's Best Interest," ibid., pp. 93–112; and Daniel Brock, "Facts and Values in the Physician–Patient Relationship," ibid., pp. 113–138.

17. Edmund D. Pellegrino, "Medical Ethics: Entering the Post-Hippocratic Era," *The Journal of the American Board of Family Practice* 1(4) (October–December 1988):230–237.

18. H. Tristram Engelhardt, Jr., and M. A. Rie, "Morality for the Medical-Industrial

Complex: A Code of Ethics for the Mass Marketing of Health Care,'' *The New England Journal of Medicine* 319(16) (October 20, 1988):1086–1089.

19. Candide's tutor in Voltaire's *Candide,* for whom all was the best in this best of all possible worlds.

20. Pellegrino and Thomasma, *For the Patient's Good.*

21. Edmund D. Pellegrino, ''Trust and Distrust in Professional Ethics,'' in Pellegrino, Veatch, and Langan (eds.), *Ethics, Trust, and the Professions,* pp. 69–85.

22. Pellegrino and Thomasma, *For the Patient's Good.*

23. Robert J. Lifton, *The Nazi Doctors: Medical Killing and the Psychology of Genocide* (New York: Basic Books, 1986); and Hugh Gallagher, *By Trust Betrayed: Patients, Physicians and the License to Kill* (New York: Holt, 1990).

24. Bernard Mandeville, *The Fable of the Bees,* ed. and intro. Philip Harth (Harmondsworth: Penguin, 1970).

25. George D. Lundberg, ''National Health Care Reform: An Aura of Inevitability Is Upon Us,'' *Journal of the American Medical Association* 265(19) (May 15, 1991):2566–2567.

26. Edmund D. Pellegrino, ''The Medical Profession as a Moral Community,'' *Bulletin of the New York Academy of Medicine* 66(3) (May–June 1990):221–232.

27. S. Woolhander and D. U. Himmelstein, ''The Deteriorating Administration of the United States Health Care System,'' *The New England Journal of Medicine* 324(18) (May 2, 1991):1253–1258.

28. George D. Lundberg, ''Fifty Hours for the Poor,'' *Journal of the American Medical Association* 262(21) (December 1, 1989):3045.

29. Engelhardt and Rie, ''Morality for Medical-Industrial Complex.''

30. Robert M. Veatch, *The Patient–Physician Relation: The Patient as Partner, Part 2.* (Bloomington: Indiana University Press, 1991), p. 63.

31. Erich Loewy, *Suffering and the Beneficent Community* (Buffalo: State University of New York Press, 1991). See also Erich Loewy, ''The Role of Suffering and Community in Clinical Ethics,'' *The Journal of Clinical Ethics* 2(2) (Summer 1991):83–89.

4

The Ends of Medicine and Its Virtues

In earlier chapters, we noted that the virtues acquire their standing within a moral community. So far, we have argued that they are interrelated with principles and moral rules within the context of that community and the wider society in which the practices of medicine occur. Since that society is constantly evolving, changes in the internal morality of the profession also occur. These changes are required by both the practice and its public expectations. Several problems arise in this scenario, however. One is that medicine should not be subject to the whims of the society in which it is found, and to its mores, without the self-critical examination brought to the discipline by medical ethics during the past thirty years. Examples of an uncritical acceptance of social mores include the Nazi physicians and their experiments, torturing of political prisoners in some countries in South America, or the use of psychiatric wards to detain and suppress political dissidents that occurred in the USSR.

A second problem arises as the culture becomes more pluralistic. When that happens, the moral basis of many of our cultural presuppositions begins to erode. What was clearly proscribed twenty years ago is now widely permitted or even encouraged. Tossed to and fro by the newest rage, individuals and subgroups within society react either by adopting the new norms and pitching out the old, by accommodation with the newer norms, or by outright rejection of "modernity." Pluralism is a good thing because it helps us reestablish and reform those cherished values that ought to persist throughout civilization, no matter what their form. The process of examination can be painful and threatening to many persons, especially those who have internalized roles, expectations, and norms. Ironically, such persons tend to be those we would call "virtuous," since they seem not to need rules by which to live, but rather act from a storehouse of experience and wisdom.

MacIntyre has thought about this problem a great deal. In his view, there are spheres of moral inquiry that have developed over the centuries. Individuals in each of these spheres or traditions have difficulty communicating or even understanding the premises of individuals in other spheres.[1] The needle hits the vinyl in considering pluralism at this juncture. For what one holds dear, another does not grant. Thus, even within medicine as a moral community, there are traditions of moral inquiry that differ profoundly with one another, so much so that it becomes difficult for the profession to police itself. Its self-regulation is abandoned to a wider and even less understanding society. This is what Robert Veatch espouses. The professions themselves demonstrate no unity of purpose. As a result, in his view, the social contract has to be renegotiated.

The third and most pressing problem, however, is that the cultural and consequent moral pluralism is constantly shifting and evolving. Not only is the amalgam changing, but the individual traditions and spheres of moral inquiry, subgroups, and ethnic diversities are also changing, in conjunction with or in apposition to the wider cultural arena.

In the midst of all this shifting sand, then, is it possible to determine certain ends of medicine that can function as the *telos* of modern medicine and the grounding of the virtues we explore? Traditionally, one looks to rules that transcend social mores and particular societies to anchor the goods of medicine or any other important human activity. We will suggest an alternate and complementary approach by looking at the doctor–patient relationship itself, as well as at the virtues that it requires in order to bring about healing.

The Ends of Medicine

A little more than a decade ago, Beauchamp and Childress published the first edition of what has since become the most influential guide to biomedical ethics.[2] They adapted W. D. Ross' notion of *prima facie* principles to the emerging field of medical ethics.[3] Today, nonmaleficence, beneficence, autonomy, and justice have become the reference tetrad *par excellence* that physicians and ethicists use to resolve ethical dilemmas and define the right conduct of physicians and patients.

As experience in the use of the four-principle framework has widened, shortcomings in its application to the clinical realities of the physician–patient relationship have begun to appear. As a result, some moral philosophers today have called for the abandonment of "principlism"[4] or its replacement by alternative theories based on virtue, feminist psychology, casuistry, or experience.[5,6]

If principles do remain integral to biomedical ethics, they will have to be more firmly grounded in the phenomena of the physician–patient relationship. One may approach this linkage in two ways. One is externally, by the application of an already developed philosophical or ethical system to the medical relationship. This is the method used by the four principles of autonomy, beneficence, nonmaleficence, and justice, whether those principles are conceived consequentially or deontologically. The second way is to examine the doctor–patient relationship with the method of philosophy (critical reflection), but without the content of a specific philosophy, in order to derive from the relationship what is required ethically and what principles and virtues combined best exemplify what is required. This is the approach via the internal morality of medicine.

This is essentially a teleological approach in the classical, not the consequentialist, sense, that is, it is oriented to the ends and purposes of the relationship. It is the degree to which decisions and actions of the moral agents—physicians and patients—approximate these ends that determines whether they are right and good.

Briefly, the ends of medicine are ultimately the restoration or improvement of health and, more proximately, to heal, that is, to cure illness and disease or, when this is not possible, to care for and help the patient to live with residual pain, discomfort, or disability. There are many decisions along the way to these ends, but in each decision there is a fusion of technical and moral elements. If it were merely a matter of technical correctness, of medical good alone, the major moral principle would be competence. But the subjects of medical decisions are humans, and humans in special states of vulnerability—anxious, in pain, and dependent upon the physician's knowledge, skill, trustworthiness, and responsible management of the power that professional status confers. Moreover, the physician offers to help and, thus, promises to the vulnerable patient to help attain the ends for which the patient seeks medical help. This implies that the physician will use her promised competence not for her own ends but for those of the patient and will, in ordinary circumstances, efface her own interests in respect for the patient; that is, she promises to serve the patient's good. But this good is more than simple medical good; it includes the patient's perception of good—material, emotional, or spiritual.

If these ends are to be achieved, the good of the patient provides the architectonic of the relationship. Beneficence becomes a requirement not of a system of philosophy applied to medicine, but of the nature of medical activity. Respect for autonomy is required to achieve the ends of medicine because to violate the patient's values is to violate his person and, therefore, a maleficent act that distorts the healing end of the relationship. Justice is a requisite duty because what we owe the patient is fidelity to the trust we elicited when we offered to help, when we invoked confidence in our willingness to act beneficently. In like fashion, the derivative obligations are mandatory if we examine the nature of the relationship. We must keep the promise we made, implicitly or explicitly, to be beneficent, to protect the patient's confidentiality (except as outlined earlier, when harm to others is at stake), and to tell the truth, since to violate any of these trusts and obligations is to go counter to the nature of the relationship itself.

In the view we take, the four principles are derived from obligations owed by physicians. These obligations, in turn, derive from the promise to provide competent help, which is at the heart of the medical relationship. The primary obligation that unifies the theory of medical ethics is beneficence—beneficence not mistakenly equated with paternalism, but beneficence in trust, beneficence that fuses respect for the person of the patient with the obligation not just to prevent or remove harm but to do good. The primary obligation is not nonmaleficence, which is a negative obligation required even by law. Beneficence requires preventing harm, removing harm, and doing good, even at some cost and risk to oneself. Thus, there is an implicit promise of some self-effacement of the physician's interests in favor of the patient's interests.

The obligations that arise from the nature of the relationship provide the theoretical grounding lacking in the approach through *prima facie* principles. Rather than principles, we can speak of obligations freely undertaken when we freely offer to help a sick person. Beneficence in trust—that is, beneficence that encompasses the patient's complete well-being, and not simply his medical well-being—becomes the ordering principle. This form of beneficence cannot obtain if we violate autonomy, justice, truth-telling, fidelity to trust, or promise keeping.

Beneficence thus becomes a principle that is also a guide to action: "So act in your relationship with your patients that your actions are directed by the good of the patient, the primary *telos* of the healing relationship." Beneficence as a principle, and the concomitant virtue of benevolence, are grounded in the humanity of the persons interacting in the medical relationship. That relationship is, as Oakeshott says of all ethics, a relationship *inter homines.*[7]

This approach has the advantage of deriving its obligations and its principles from real phenomena of the real world of clinical medicine. It reverses the usual way philosophy is used to determine medical ethics. Rather than taking principles already formulated in an ethical theory—consequentialist, utilitarian, or deontological—it begins with the phenomena peculiar to the activity in question and examines them philosophically—that is, critically, formally, systematically, in terms of the human realities they exemplify. It may indeed happen, as in the present inquiry, that the results are similar to those of the four-principle approach. But the principles are grounded in a more systematic use of theory; its principles flow from obligations grounded in the special character of the medical relationship. They become more than a checklist of considerations for ethical discourse. They have a moral binding power grounded firmly in clinical realities.

Clearly, the teleological approach suggested here does not, by itself, constitute a complete system of medical ethics. To do so, it would also have to link obligations and its primary principles to virtue ethics and incorporate insights from casuistry, moral psychology, and experiential ethical systems. In the final part of the book, we discuss the possibility of an integral medical ethics that would ideally combine all these features.

The four-principle approach does have theoretical and practical inadequacies. However, it should not be abandoned because it still has much to offer. Its shortcomings can be remedied. The one area of refinement we have suggested is a closer and firmer grounding in the **physician–patient relationship**. Another area, which is examined only partially in the rest of the book, is to incorporate insights from experience, moral psychology, casuistry, and virtue theories. In the years ahead, such efforts could produce a more complete theory and practice of medical ethics, provided that the theory is firmly situated in the central pediment of all biomedical ethics, the physician–patient relationship.

Autonomy and the Models of the Physician–Patient Relationship

Nothing in medical ethics has changed so dramatically and drastically in the last quarter century as the standards of ethical conduct governing the relationship between physicians and patients. In that time, the center of gravity of clinical decision-making has shifted almost completely from the physician to the patient. The traditional benign and respected image of the physician as both moral and technical authority has been replaced by the physician as protector, facilitator, and advocate for the self-determination of the patient. Now every facet of care, from the choice among preferred treatments to the request not to be resuscitated, and even for active euthanasia and assisted suicide, is construed as a moral and civil right with which doctors in good conscience are expected to comply.

This metamorphosis has been most evident and most advanced in the United States. But the sociopolitical and cultural forces that have nurtured such a drastic change are effecting similar transformations in almost every country of the world. Among these forces are the actualization of participatory democracy, the increasing moral pluralism and moral heterogeneity of modern society, expansion of public education by the media, the weakening of religion as an ultimate source of morality, a general mistrust of the exercise of authority in all spheres of life, and, of course, the unprecedented expansion of medical power through technology.

Not the least of the forces effecting change has been the entry of the professional philosopher into the study of medical ethics. Curiously, philosophers historically paid little formal attention to the ethics of medicine. To be sure, there were "philosophical" reflections by physicians on the nature of medicine and medical ethics, but this was philosophy only in the loosest sense. Until the mid-1960s, professional philosophers paid little formal attention to medical ethics.

This changed when medical ethics first came under serious philosophical scrutiny. Surely the most influential thrust in this direction was Beauchamp and Childress' *Principles of Bioethics,* first published in 1978, in which the four-principle approach around which this whole book is organized was first introduced.[8] This book added the reinforcement of formal analysis to the more inchoate stirrings of social change that had already weakened the pediments of the traditional Hippocratic model of the physician–patient relationship. In its place, a variety of autonomy-based models have gained preeminence.

Given the confluence of forces we mentioned above as characteristic of modern democratic, secular, morally heterogeneous societies, the principle of autonomy has had understandable worldwide appeal both inside and outside medicine. Autonomy, self-governance, and the right to privacy have become symbols of resistance to the misuse of authority by professionals, institutions, and governments. Respect for autonomy seeks to balance the enormous power of expert knowledge that figures so prominently in private and public decisions in industrialized, technologically oriented societies. Autonomy calls for protection of the moral and personal values of each individual and, thus, of the integrity of the person.

Autonomy has particular appeal in medical relationships. It counters the historical dominance of benign authoritarianism or paternalism in the traditional ethics of medicine. It ensures that patients may choose among treatment alternatives, accept or reject any of them, and thus retain control over some of the most intimate and personal decisions in their lives. Respect for autonomy also protects patients against submergence of their moral values and beliefs. In morally diverse societies where physicians and patients may have markedly different cultural, ethnic, and religious origins, observance of this facet of autonomy is especially and justifiably cherished.

The assertion of autonomy in medical ethics has been salubrious on the whole. It has become a powerful and increasingly effective deterrent to abuses of physicians' power. It has served particularly well in placing the ultimate control of decisions at the beginning and end of life more fully under the control of the patient. It is the driving force behind judicial opinions and legislation that confirm the legal rights of patients to make their own decisions and to make use of advance directives to ensure control of decisions if competence to do so is lost in the course of an illness.

The emphasis on autonomy has also fostered the emergence of several models of the physician–patient relationship sharply divergent from traditional models.[9] Two examples are the consumer model and the negotiated contract model.

In the consumer model, health care is view as a commodity or service, like any other commodity, to be purchased in the marketplace on the consumer's terms, that is, in terms of his or her personal assessment of alternative modes of treatment, their cost, benefits, and risks. The physician is a provider whose task is to provide reliable information and perhaps to advise, but not to interject his or her own values. The patient's values must predominate. The physician's moral obligations are to inform, to perform with competence, and to protect and enhance the patient's capabilities for self-determination.

In the negotiated contract model, physician and patient discuss their relative values in advance—those related to health and those related to moral values in general. As in the consumer model, physician and patient are both autonomous persons entering a contract, but in the negotiated model, the details of the contract are more intensively examined before any medical relationship begins. Moreover, the nature of the relationship is determinable only by the contracting parties. In essence, they alone must determine what conduct is expected, so that the ethics of the relationship varies with the ethics of the contracting parties. In this view, the notion of a universally applicable set of ethical principles beyond autonomy is irrelevant. Physician and patient may pursue any course they wish, provided that it is mutually agreed upon. But the fact that this is agreed upon is no concern of third parties. It might include active euthanasia, assisted suicide, or an advance directive that calls for involuntary or nonvoluntary euthanasia.

These two examples of autonomy-driven models of the doctor–patient relationship make the relationship largely instrumental and procedural. They are legalistic in spirit, and the ethic they engender is one of minimal personal commitment and trust. Indeed, they are based more on distrust than on trust. They are destructive also of the idea of a common medical morality, since the participants give medical ethics any meaning they choose. The only ethical failure is the failure to abide by a prearranged contract.

While these autonomy-inspired models seem to protect the patient's right of self-determination, on closer inspection they are also, in considerable measure, illusory and even dangerous to both parties. First, they neglect the fact that the physician and patient are not Lockean free agents equal in bargaining power. The patient is vulnerable, since she is the one in need of help, has not the power to heal herself, and is in pain, anxious, frightened, and perhaps distressed. It is hard to imagine a valid contract in which one party is so dependent upon the other for the information necessary to a choice and upon the competence of the other to carry out the choice once it is made.

Autonomy-based models thus seem oblivious to the incontestable fact of physician power, a power that arises from several sources. There is the *de facto* power just mentioned, which derives from the fact of illness itself. But there is also the power of the physician's personality or charisma, which operates in subtle ways often inapparent to both physician and patient but is nonetheless a powerful force in shaping even the independently minded patient's decisions. Finally, there is the force of social sanction of medicine and its monopoly of medical knowledge, which operate regardless of the details of a negotiated contract.

The realities of these forms of "Aesculapian power" make it amply evident that the desire to limit trust in the physician that lies behind the autonomy models is often deceptive. There is no way to circumvent the physician's character or her construal of what autonomy means in actual practice. In fact, to execute a contract is to send a signal of distrust of the physician and to put her on her guard. As a result, she might restrain her inclination to be beneficent when the clinical situation changes in ways that could not have been anticipated. In any case, there is no evidence that a relationship based on mistrust is any more protective of patient autonomy than one based on trust, that is, on a covenant rather that a contract.[10]

The deficiencies of autonomy-based models of the physician–patient relationship do not, of course, vitiate the validity of autonomy as a moral principle. There is no question that the centuries-old neglect of the role of the patient in decisions that affect him is not, and was not, morally defensible even if it was socially tolerable. Respect for the patient's self-determination, and thus for the integrity of the person, is a moral requirement in all human relationships, especially in those like medicine, in which there is a *de facto* imbalance of power. For this reason, after we complete our exploration of the virtues in medicine in Part II, we will turn again to a discussion of respect for persons and the role of autonomy within the virtue of benevolence. What the deficiencies of the models that try to optimize autonomy reveal is not that autonomy is to be abandoned, but that absolutization is morally perilous. If autonomy itself is to be safeguarded, its expression must be more closely related to the other major principles of beneficence and justice, as well as to theories of medical ethics that are not principle-based, but rather arise from virtues and experience.

Conflicts of Autonomy with Beneficence

A second consequence of the autonomy movement is the degree to which patient self-determination is set in polar opposition to beneficence. This emerges clearly in Beauchamp's book with L. B. McCullough.[11] Here beneficence is erroneously equated with paternalism. The case examples used to illustrate the conceptual content of the text choices are framed almost exclusively as conflicts between beneficence and autonomy. Several misconceptions arise as a result. This is particularly unfortunate from the point of view of our philosophy of medicine, since beneficence itself is subsumed under the virtue of justice in the sense that it is owed to the patient from the healing end of medicine. Let us clear up some points of confusion at the outset.

First of all, beneficence and paternalism are not synonymous. Paternalism (or maternalism) assumes that the physician knows better than the patient what is in the patient's best interests, or that even a mentally competent patient cannot possibly know enough about the choices to be able to make intelligent decisions. Or, less benignly, the physician may assume that it is her prerogative as the privileged proprietor of medical knowledge and skill to dispense it as she sees fit, without the patient's interference.

Paternalism, whether benignly intended or not, cannot be beneficent in any true sense of that word. Beneficence and its corollary, nonmaleficence, require acting to advance the patient's interests, or at least not harming them. It is difficult to see how violating the patient's own perception of his welfare can be a beneficent act. Paternalism is obviously in a polar relationship with autonomy, but it is diametrically opposed to beneficence and nonmaleficence as well.

True beneficence, on the other hand, seeks the good of the patient. That good is a compound idea consisting of an ascending hierarchy: (1) what is medically good, that is, restoration of physiological functioning and emotional balance; (2) what is defined as good by the patient in terms of his perception of his own good; (3) what is good for humans as humans and members of the human community; and (4) what is good for humans as spiritual beings.[12]

In this hierarchical order, autonomy is a good of humans as humans. Without freedom and the capacity to make choices about our own lives, to be responsible for those choices, and to carry out a life plan, we cannot express our humanity fully. To violate or impede a patient's autonomy is a maleficent act. To facilitate, enhance, and restore the capability for self-governance is a beneficent act. Beneficence and respect for persons, which are the moral foundation for autonomy, are therefore congruent, and it is a misconception to see them as antithetical, as some interpreters of the four principles do. Later we will suggest an alternative perspective on the four principles that may help to resolve potential conflicts between autonomy and beneficence, as well as the potential conflict with justice, to be examined in Chapter 7.

"Tuning" the Four Principles Philosophically and Clinically

To bring the four-principle approach into closer congruence with some of the realities of clinical decision-making and the virtues of medicine, we need to examine at least three questions: (1) How are conflicts between *prima facie* principles to be resolved? (2) How may other sources of ethical insight be incorporated? (3) What, finally, should be the relationship of formal philosophy to medical ethics?

The Conflict Between Prima Facie Principles

The framework of *prima facie* principles has unquestionably advanced the quality of ethical decision-making at the bedside. Its utility must not be lost in the current zeal for replacing it with alternative approaches that have their own inherent difficulties. The four principles have put the whole process of moral decision making on a more orderly, less idiosyncratic, and more explicit basis. They have raised sensitivities to ethical issues among all health care workers, patients, and their families. The general moral precepts of the Hippocratic ethics have been fleshed out where they have been deficient and provided with philosophical grounding where this has been lacking. Principle-based ethics has also provided a *lingua franca* for communication among physicians and ethicists, whose moral presuppositions might otherwise have been incommensurable with one another.

It would be a retrogressive step indeed to drop the principles and return to some simplistic conviction of the sufficiency of the Hippocratic Oath, to which many physicians subscribe. Equally unsatisfactory would be a too ready acquiescence to the arguments of the antiprinciplists, who would substitute important but insufficient bases for medical ethics drawn from virtue, feminist, or experiential systems. These alternatives, valuable as they are, also lead to subjectivism, emotivism, and egoism, the major dangers to which non-principle-based approaches are susceptible.

This is not to deny a central difficulty in the design of the system of *prima facie* principles. If these principles are to be honored, unless there is an overwhelming reason not to do so, what constitutes an overwhelming reason? Is the justification for overriding made in terms of some other *prima facie* principle or some special circumstance? If it is another *prima facie* principle, then we face the problem of one principle having greater moral weight than another. There is no formal mechanism or convincing argument that would grant trumping privileges to one principle over another.

Clearly, prima facie principles cannot be used to resolve conflicts among *prima facie* principles unless some external ordering mechanism is adduced, as suggested in the prior discussion of the autonomy–beneficence polarity. Could the trumping justification, then, simply be the circumstances? If this were the case, the circumstances themselves would take on the moral force of a *prima facie* principle, or they would have to be justified by one of the *prima facie* principles—but which one?

Any and all of these attempts to resolve the conflict between *prima facie* principles must eventually pit one *prima facie* principle against another. This leads to the logical error of begging the question or circular reasoning. If this is so, then some resolution must be sought beyond *prima facie* principles, and this could come about in one of five ways: (1) abandon principlism altogether in favor of some alternate theory like virtue, experience, or feminist psychology; (2) retain principlism, but supplement it by insights from other ethical theories; (3) ground principlism more fully in the phenomena of the doctor–patient relationship; (4) some combination of options 2 and 3; or (5) retain the four-principle approach without emendation.

From what we have shown thus far, it is clear that options 1 and 5 are not adequate in the face of the practical and theoretical complexities described here. Option 4 seems the most promising, and this option will be examined briefly here, leaving to other parts of the book its more extended development.

Principlism has sustained its most radical criticism in the work of Clouser and Gert and others.[13,14] These authors point out what they take to be fundamental conceptual flaws in principlism as exemplified specifically in the work of Frankena[15] and Beauchamp and Childress. Clouser and Gert assert that principlism "lacks systematic unity and thus creates both practical and theoretical problems. Since there is no moral theory that ties 'principles' together, there is no unified guide to action which generates clear, coherent, comprehensive, and specific rules for action nor any justification of those rules."[16] In Clouser and Gert's view, these inadequacies lead to relativism, since principles seem to stand free of any grounding and since they may conflict with each other without offering a path to resolution. Similar criticisms can be found in the articles by Brody[17] and Green.[18] Criticism of another kind comes from the protagonists of virtue theory, feminist psychology, casuistry, or ethics as narrative, experiential, or existential phenomena. Space limitations prohibit serious examination of these alternatives. However, they share the perceptions that principle-based ethics is too abstract, too removed from the moral and psychological realities of actual people making actual choices, and too male-oriented in its psychology and reasoning. They also aver that principlism ignores the character, gender, life stories, and cultural identity of moral agents. In this view, ethics is more than a technical exercise drawing clear conclusions from clear premises. It is a personal act nuanced in a variety of subtle ways that principles do not touch. As Oakeshott puts it, "moral conduct is art, not nature."[19]

One may agree that there is substance in each of these criticisms of principle-based ethics without also agreeing that they do away with principles or are themselves fully adequate replacements. It is too soon to know how, and to what extent, they will modify the four-principle approach. The likelihood is that they will enrich and refine principle-based ethics but not replace it.[20,21] It seems unclear that a unifying theory of biomedical ethics will need to link principles with insights from these other sources. This is the most serious conceptual task biomedical ethics faces in the immediate future.

Conclusion

As we have mentioned, a traditional method of approaching moral and social pluralism is to find some absolute values that somehow transcend a culture. We suspect that the effort to develop principles of biomedical ethics stems in part from this tendency. Even though, at root, each person, each case, and each event is unique, there are common features that help us resolve moral dilemmas more efficiently as we gain experience. From these common features evolve moral rules, norms, standards, and principles.

In this final propaedeutic chapter, we have suggested an alternative approach to the problem of pluralism. Rather than look solely to moral principles, one should also examine the virtues that have spanned the history of medicine to this day. These virtues lock into the healing ends of medicine, which also have not changed to a great extent over the centuries. Although with new technologies and new methods of delivery the ends are constantly being reinterpreted, the bond of healing in the doctor–patient relationship is still the ultimate goal of the profession. If it is not, something is askew. Its purpose is lost. By definition, it is no longer medicine.

We are now ready to examine some of these virtues in detail in the next section of the book. Once again, a reminder: we have had to be selective about the virtues we examine. Both space and time limit this examination. Among those virtues left out, and deserving of scrutiny, are **intellectual honesty, humility**, and **therapeutic parsimony**.

Notes

1. Alasdair C. MacIntyre, *Three Rival Versions of Moral Enquiry: Encyclopedia, Geneology, and Tradition* (Notre Dame, IN: University of Notre Dame Press, 1990).

2. Tom L. Beauchamp and James F. Childress, *Principles of Biomedical Ethics,* 3d ed. (New York: Oxford University Press, 1989).

3. W. D. Ross, *The Foundations of Ethics* (Oxford: Clarendon Press, 1939).

4. K. Danner Clouser and Bernard Gert, "A Critique of Principlism," *Journal of Medicine and Philosophy* 15(2) (April 1990):219–236.

5. Carol Gilligan, *In a Different Voice: Psychological Theory and Women's Development* (Cambridge, MA: Harvard University Press, 1982).

6. James F. Drane, *Becoming a Good Doctor: The Place of Virtue and Character in Medical Ethics* (Kansas City, MO: Sheed and Ward, 1988).

7. Michael J. Oakeshott, *"Rationalism in Politics" and Other Essays* (New York: Basic Books, 1962).

8. Beauchamp and Childress, *Principles.*

9. Ezekial J. Emanuel and Linda Emanuel, "Four Models of the Physician–Patient Relationship," *Journal of the American Medical Association* 267(16) (April 22/29, 1992):2221–2226.

10. William F. May, *The Physician's Covenant* (Philadelphia: Westminster Press, 1983).

11. Tom L. Beauchamp and Laurence B. McCullough, *Medical Ethics: The Moral Responsibilities of Physicians* (Englewood Cliffs, NJ: Prentice-Hall, 1984).

12. Edmund D. Pellegrino and David C. Thomasma, *For the Patient's Good: The Restoration of Beneficence in Health Care* (New York: Oxford University Press, 1988).

13. Clouser and Gert, "Critique."

14. Ronald M. Green, "Method in Bioethics: A Troubled Assessment," *Journal of Medicine and Philosophy* 15(2) (April 1990):179–197.

15. William K. Frankena, *Ethics* (Englewood Cliffs, NJ: Prentice-Hall, 1973).

16. Clouser and Gert, "Critique," p. 227.

17. Baruch A. Brody, "Quality of Scholarship in Bioethics," *Journal of Medicine and Philosophy* 15(2) (April 1990):161–178.

18. Green, "Method in Bioethics."

19. Oakeshott, *"Rationalism in Politics,"* p. 296.

20. Alisa L. Carse, "The Voice of Care: Implications for Bioethical Education," *Journal of Medicine and Philosophy* 16(1) (February 1991):5–28.

21. Albert R. Jonsen and Stephen E. Toulmin, *The Abuse of Casuistry: A History of Moral Reasoning* (Los Angeles: University of California Press, 1988).

6. See Stephen L. Daniel (Guest Ed.), "Interpretation in Medicine," *Theoretical Medicine* 11 (1) (March 1990), entire issue.

7. Plato, *Lesser Hippias,* in *The Dialogues of Plato,* trans. B. Jowett, intro. by Raphael Demos (New York: Random House, 1937), pp. 715–729.

8. Generally, for the most part true, ethical principles before the age of reason were not considered to be *a priori* with metaphysical, but rather with ethical, certitude. Exception were admitted in principle; see MacIntyre, *After Virtue.*

9. St. Thomas Aquinas, *Summa Theologiae,* 2, 2ae, qq. 47–48.

10. St. Thomas Aquinas, *Summa Theologiae,* 1, 2ae, q. 57, a. 4.

11. R. M. Hare, *Freedom and Reason* (New York: Oxford-Clarendon Press, 1965), pp. 3–37.

12. St. Thomas Aquinas, *Summa Theologiae,* 1, 2ae, qq. 9–10; q. 18.

13. *Ibid.* qq. 65–67; 2, 2ae, qq. 47–51.

14. Etienne Gilson, *Moral Values and the Moral Life: The Ethical Theory of St. Thomas Aquinas* (Hamden, CT: Shoe String Press, 1961).

15. David Hume, *An Enquiry Concerning the Principles of Morals,* ed. J. B. Schneewind (Indianapolis: Hackett, 1960), pp. 85, n. 30.

16. David Hume, *A Treatise of Human Nature,* ed. L. A. Selby-Bigge (New York: Oxford-Clarendon Press, 1978), p. 477.

17. V. M. Hope, *Virtue in Consensus: The Moral Philosophies of Hutcheson, Hume and Adam Smith* (New York: Oxford-Clarendon Press, 1989), p. 2.

18. Beauchamp and Childress, *Principles,* p. 375.

19. Ibid.

20. Ibid., p. 379.

21. Ibid., p. 380.

22. Ibid., p. 381.

23. Pellegrino and Thomasma, *For the Patient's Good: Toward the Restoration of Beneficence in Health Care* (New York: Oxford University Press, 1988).

24. Glenn C. Graber and David C. Thomasma, *Theory and Practice in Medical Ethics* (New York: Continuum, 1989), pp. 155–172.

25. Gregory Pence, *Ethical Options in Medicine* (Oradell, N.J.: Medical Economics, 1980), pp. 17ff.

26. Stan Sesser, "A Reporter at Large: A Nation of Contradictions," *The New Yorker* 67(47) (January 13, 1992):37–68, p. 54.

27. Henry K. Beecher, "Tentative Statement Outlining the Philosophy and Ethical Principles Governing the Conduct of Research on Human Beings at the Harvard Medical School," *Experimentation with Human Beings,* ed. Jay Katz (New York: Russell Sage Foundation, 1972), p. 849.

28. Franz Ingelfinger, "Arrogance," *New England Journal of Medicine* 303(26) (December 25 1980):1507–1511.

29. Bernard Lonergan, *Insight: A Study of Human Understanding* (San Francisco: Harper & Row, 1978), p. 388.

30. Ibid.

31. Ibid., p. 389.

32. See note 8.

33. Alasdair MacIntyre, *Three Rival Versions of Moral Enquiry: Encyclopedia, Genealogy, and Tradition* (Notre Dame, IN: University of Notre Dame Press, 1990), p. 139.

34. Michael Oakeshott, *"Rationalism in Politics" and Other Essays* (Indianapolis: Liberty Press, 1991), p. 295.

II

THE VIRTUES IN MEDICINE

> The moral life is a life *inter-homines*.
>
> MICHAEL OAKESHOTT

Alasdair MacIntyre has stressed repeatedly that the interrelation of professional virtues and principles relies upon the grounding of both in the community and its values. As he says of the "communal" and moral rules:

> Detach them [the moral rules] from their place in defining and constituting a whole way of life and they become nothing but a set of arbitrary prohibitions, as they too often became in later periods. To possess or both moral energy and the moral life is then to progress in understanding all the various aspects of that life, rules, precepts, virtues, passions, actions as parts of a single whole.

It is therefore important in our line of argument to consider the ways in which medicine itself functions as the moral community that both shapes the ends of the moral life of those who practice health care healing and the means by which these are concretized in their virtuous actions.

Challenges in Professional Ethics

The most crucial dilemmas of medical ethics today are not those arising from medicine's scientific progress. They are dilemmas of professional ethics, those that go to the heart of what it is to be a physician. In these matters, medicine faces its own ethical choice. It must reconcile two competing orders — one based on the primacy of its covenant with patients and the other based on the ethos of self-interest. Think about just most of the major challenges to this tension between self-interest and altruism: whether to disclose one's HIV-positive status, having an economic interest in an MRI unit to which one refers patients, whether there is a duty to treat all patients who request care, the problem of health care for the poor and one's obligations in this regard, the reform of the health care system, conflicts about requests for public policy for physician-assisted suicide, integrity in biomedical research, the medical-industrial complex, physicians' incentives as gatekeepers to keep costs down, and many others. Each of these dilemmas, although occasioned by technology, arises from changing roles of the profession in response to public and

5

Fidelity to Trust

Ademantus, I wonder men dare trust themselves with men.
TIMON OF ATHENS, 1, 2, 43

Trust is ineradicable in human relationships. Without it we could not live in society or attain even the rudiments of a fulfilling life. Without trust we could not anticipate the future, and we would therefore be paralyzed into inaction. Yet to trust and entrust is to become vulnerable and dependent on the good will and motivations of those we trust. Trust, ineradicable as it is, is also always problematic.

Trust is most problematic when we are in states of special dependence—in illness, old age, or infancy or when we are in need of healing, justice, spiritual help, or learning. This is the situation in our relationships with the professions that circumstances force us to trust. We are forced to trust professionals if we wish access to their knowledge and skill. We need the help of doctors, lawyers, ministers, rabbis, priests, chaplains, or teachers to surmount or cope with our most pressing human needs. We must depend on their fidelity to trust and their desire to protect rather than exploit our vulnerability.

This ineradicability of trust has been a generative force in professional ethics for a long time. To be sure, there have always been professionals who violated trust, but they were the moral renegades and pariahs. Recently the central place of trust in professional ethics been seriously doubted or attacked, not only as an illusion but even as a radical impossibility.[1] Indeed, what amounts to an ethics of distrust has been gathering force. It would place tighter restraints on professionals or eliminate the need for trust entirely. To this end, alternatives to trust in the ethics of the professions are proposed—reducing professional relationships to contracts, or appointing ombudsmen or other intermediaries to monitor the advice and actions of professionals.

Without depreciating the reality of the factors that generate the distrust, arguments for an ethic of distrust are flawed empirically, phenomenologically, and conceptually. In the professional realm, the ethics of distrust is perilous, self-defeating, and ultimately impossible in practice. It is sounder to acknowledge the ineradicability of trust and to restructure the ethics of the professions even more solidly on this foundation. This restructuring in no way necessitates the subjugation of patient choice to the professional's value system or a blunting of the salubrious move toward an ethics of patient autonomy and participation.

To advance the ethics of trust against the ethics of distrust, we shall first examine the phenomenon of trust, both in general and in the professional context. Then we shall examine the rise of the ethics of distrust and its inherent fallacies, and finally the inescapable obligations that the ineradicability of trust imposes on professionals and on patients as well.

The Phenomenology of Trust

Trust as a General Phenomenon in All Human Relationships

Despite its ubiquity in human affairs, trust has been examined only tangentially by philosophers, although it is a central virtue in Christian ethics. It has yet to receive extended and formal philosophical analysis. Recent writers have begun such an inquiry from different points of view and with different conceptual formulations.

Bernard Barber, a sociologist, identifies trust with the expectation that social actors will observe three conditions: (1) they will act within a persistent moral order, (2) they will perform their technical roles competently, and (3) roles that require a special concern for others, such as the fiduciary role, will be faithfully fulfilled.[2] So far as professions go, Barber sees three distinctive characteristics that have a special bearing on trust: (1) their possession of powerful knowledge, (2) the autonomy necessary to their practice and, (3) their fiduciary obligation to individuals and society.[3] Barber's analysis is largely descriptive, and it treats the moral foundations of trust only indirectly.

Niklas Luhmann, another sociologist, provides a much more sophisticated and detailed account of trust and distrust. His account offers valuable insights into the ineradicability of trust and its functions in complex societies. Luhmann's hypothesis is that trust is associated with "reduction of complexity," more specifically with the complexity that enters the world as a consequence of the freedom of other human beings.[4] By trusting, we remove the burden and impediment of complexity:

> Trust then is the generalized expectation that another will handle his freedom, his disturbing potential for diverse action in keeping with his personality, or rather in keeping with the personality which he has presented and made socially visible. He who stands by what he has consciously or unconsciously allowed to be known about himself is worthy of trust.[5]

While trust aims to reduce complexity, it also unavoidably involves contingency. Some persons attempt to avoid contingency by distrust—by withdrawing confidence in the expectation that the person trusted will not abuse that confidence. But, at the same time, distrust reduces the range of possible human relationships and thus the fulfillment one can attain in life. Obviously, all but the most reclusive humans can or would want to rule their lives by trust rather than distrust.

Luhmann seeks a possible way out of the risks inherent in trust by transferring trust from person-to-person relationships to "system trust." Confidence is placed in institutional and social structures to reduce complexity by the restraints they impose on individuals who function within them. This seems a highly problematic solution given that the relationships between individuals and institutions are neither less notably complex nor more notably reliable than person-to-person relationships.

Annette Baier has undertaken the ambitious task of a formal inquiry into the nature of trust, a subject that has been neglected in philosophical discourse. As she points out, except for Hume's focus on promise and contract, and trust in God emphasized by theologians, most writers have given only tangential attention to this subject.

Baier defines trust as "reliance on others' competence and willingness to look after, rather than harm, the things one cares about which are entrusted to their care."[6] She defines different kinds of trust relationships: the differences between promise, contracts, and trust, and the conditions that make trust "morally decent." She emphasizes the vulnerability involved in trusting another person, the indispensability and dangers of discretionary power given the one trusted, and the necessity of confidence that the trusting person's vulnerability will not be exploited, even if the one trusted person has motives for doing so. Baier's inquiry illustrates the complexity of trust and the need for a better understanding of the philosophical (and, by extension, theological) foundations for morally valid trust relationships. Her account notes some of the special qualities of the professional relationship. Although she does not examine these in detail, she provides insights into the general phenomena that are relevant to any consideration of the special features of relationships with professionals.

Most construals of trust involve several elements, the strength and combinations of which vary with the nature of the relationship between the person trusted and the person trusting. The first element is confidence that expectations of fidelity to what is entrusted will be fulfilled. Second is the sense that the person trusted has explicitly or implicitly made a promise to act well with respect to the interests of the person trusted. Third is the belief that discretionary latitude of certain proportions is necessary if trust is to be fulfilled, and that the one trusted will use it well, assuming neither too much nor too little. Fourth is the congruence of understanding on these first three elements between the one trusting and the one trusted. Finally, underlying all of these aspects is an act of faith in the benevolence and good character of the one trusted. Each of these five elements takes on special meaning in the context of relationships with professionals.

Trust in Relationships with Professionals

Like other human relationships, our relationships with professionals ineradicably involve trust. Here trust has special moral dimensions that are the foundation for professional ethics, what Barber has called "fiduciary relationships."[7] Trust in the helping professions—medicine, law, ministry, and teaching—has many features in common. Each relationship deserves examination in its own right, but only one will be examined here. The medical relationship will serve to illustrate the way trust shapes the ethical relationships between patients and physicians, and by analogy the relationships between lawyers and clients, clergy and parishioners, and teachers and students.

People seek out physicians when some adverse sign or symptom threatens their conception of their health sufficiently to impel them to seek expert advice. As soon as persons decide they need help, they become patients—they bear a burden of anxiety, pain, or suffering. To seek professional help is to trust that physicians possess the capacity to help and heal. From the very first moment, the patient performs an act of trust: first, in the existence and utility of medical knowledge itself, and then in its possession by the one who is being consulted. Trust at this initial level is more like what Baier calls "reliance," the kind of trust we place in airline pilots, firemen, or policemen—a trust inspired less by the person than by the common recognition of a defined social role.[8] It is an expression of general confidence somewhat akin to Luhmann's "system trust."

We do not usually interview the pilot who is to take us over the ocean or worry about his motives or self-interest. Presumably he wishes to make as safe a crossing as we. The pilot's competence is vital, and his discretionary powers in flight are well nigh absolute. But his involvement with us as persons is remote. Our trust in him is situated in trust in the system more than in the individual.

If we take medical relationships as our paradigm case, we recognize a certain amount of trust in the system of education, credentialing, and the processes of licensure. But the intimacy, specificity, and personal nature of relationships with physicians compel us to be more concerned with personal qualities—with personality, but most of all with character.[9] Except in emergencies, at the earliest stages of a medical relationship, we are freer than we are in the choice of our pilot. We can consult other physicians and former patients and check credentials, as well as do research on the advice we receive. Here the system can serve to establish or reinforce trust.

But before we engage this presumably competent physician, we are interested in much more. We expect to open the most private domains of our bodies, minds, and social and family relationships to her probing gaze. Our vices, foibles, and weaknesses will be exposed to a stranger. Even our living and dying will engage her attention and invite her counsel. This is not at all like our trust in the pilot. The system cannot provide the reassurance we may want. Ultimately, we must place our trust in the person of the physician. We want someone who knows about us, treats us non-judgmentally, and is concerned with our welfare. We want someone who will use the discretionary latitude our care requires with circumspection— neither intruding nor presuming too much nor undertaking too little. We must be able to trust her to do what she is trusted to do, that is, to serve the healing purposes for which we have given our trust in the first place.

We must trust also that our vulnerability will not be exploited for power, profit, prestige, or pleasure. The physician's or lawyer's superior knowledge and skill foreordain inequality in the relationship. Even if we are physicians or lawyers ourselves, our capacity for objectivity is compromised when we are ill or named in a lawsuit. We know we can be deceived or led to the choice the lawyer or physician wants by the way he selects the facts about what can be done to help us. We can, to be sure, elicit other opinions, read for ourselves about our illnesses, or speak to other patients. But ultimately, we must decide not only what we should do, but who will do it. What we want and what the doctor prescribes may be in conflict. We have to choose between our own judgment and that of someone we trust to have knowledge and a commitment to our well-being.

No professional can function properly without discretionary latitude. The more discretionary latitude we permit our professionals, the more vulnerable we become. Yet to limit that latitude is to limit the capacity for good as much as it may limit the capacity for harm. When all is said and done, we cannot anticipate every contingency even in a disease we understand well. Chronically ill patients often understand their illnesses better than physicians. Yet they can also be distressingly misinformed. At some point, even our intimate knowledge of our needs must be translated into action. That action will be taken by another person—the physician, lawyer, or clergy on whom we are forced to depend if our goals are to be realized.

We can consult different authorities about our medical, legal, or spiritual problems. We may evaluate their logic, the evidence they adduce, or their compatibility with our personal values. Yet when there are differences among experts, we must choose among them. And when we do, we really are choosing the professional we think we can trust to carry out our wishes and respect our values. Even then, every iota of our evaluation of our own situation may not be perfectly congruent with that of our physician, lawyer, or pastor.

We cannot subject every suggestion, recommendation, or counsel to the same intensive process of investigation for logical credibility. Even the most skeptical and distrusting patient would be exhausted by such an effort. At some point, we must trust in our mutual understanding of what is in the sick person's interests. One might argue that only serious decisions need to be thoroughly examined. But what constitutes a serious decision? To answer this question, the patient needs information, again from a source that can be trusted. We can consult other experts or textbooks of medicine. But, once again, how does one choose among conflicting opinions? How does the patient deal with the fact that textbooks and articles are quickly out-of-date? A competent clinician will usually be more closely attuned to the rapidity of changes in the state of the art.

Let us suppose that a physician has been chosen because his opinion and recommendation after our investigations seem more credible than his colleague's. We still have the question of skill in carrying out the recommendations. How does one check on skill? Some patients seek out a surgeon's morbidity and mortality statistics or the opinions of her peers. Here we must trust the surgeon's honesty in reporting or the objectivity of her peers. We would find out that all surgeons have a certain irreducible mortality and morbidity. We must trust that the one we have chosen will have the skill requisite for a beneficial outcome.

Even the most distrustful and skeptical patient must at some point confront the fact that the physician is the final pathway through which all things medical must funnel. It is the physician who writes the orders, performs the procedure, and interprets the recommendations of other health professionals. The physician is a *de facto* gatekeeper who we trust to be the patient's advocate, and not simply an instrument of social, institutional, or fiscal policies.[10] Depending on his character and fidelity of trust, he may treat the patient as a statistical entity or he may be the patient's last protection against the system. These contingencies are all exacerbated by the fact that trust in professional relationships is forced since it is trust generated by our need for help. When we need a doctor, lawyer, or pastor, we have no choice but to trust someone, though we might prefer to trust none.

Advance directives, like living wills, are a good example of attempts to supplant trust by contractual agreement. They seek to make the wishes of patients explicit to family and physician, particularly regarding terminal care. Morally and legally, they have the same force as a competent patient's decision. They can settle or avoid disputes about what is in the patient's best interests. They also forewarn the physician who may choose not to enter the relationship if she disagrees with the patient's values.

But advance directives cannot specify every detail and every contingency. They are open to interpretation, particularly the physician's or family's understanding of what the patient meant by "ordinary" or "extraordinary" measures or doing "everything possible."

If living wills are written too tightly, they limit the physician's discretionary latitude in ways the patient might not really want. If written too broadly, they leave too much room for dispute and presumption. Living wills must be implemented through human agency. Those who write them must trust that those who eventually carry out their wishes will act out of good will. In short, living wills cannot supplant trust because their execution depends on it. For these reasons, a durable power of attorney for health care is a better instrument, since it substitutes for written instructions verbal ones to an individual empowered to work with physicians on behalf of the patient when the patient becomes incompetent. A dialogical relationship is much better than a physician–paper one, since one's course of illness resembles a drama in which changes may take place daily.

Replacing trust relationships by contracts for care is equally dependent upon trust. Contracts can diminish the risk of frustration of the patient's will, but again, they are based on trust that the things agreed to will, in fact, be performed. Contracts cannot envision all contingencies. They must allow discretionary latitude to the professional or they are self-defeating.

Moreover, the whole concept of a contract between someone who is ill, in need of justice, or worried about salvation and the professional who can help meet those needs is illusory.[11] Contracts are negotiated between equals or near-equals. This is simply not the case in relationships with doctors, lawyers, or clergy and chaplains. Contracts must trust also that there is understanding of mutual interest beyond the phraseology of the contract. The same words too often carry different meanings. The frequency with which breach of contract is alleged is ample testimony that there is implicit trust even in the most explicitly worded agreement. The contract, therefore, implies that the competent contractor (the physician in this case) guarantees that he will pay attention, not only to the meanings of the contract but also to the imbalanced relationship created by the dynamics of illness and dependency.[12]

It is clear from the empirical and conceptual points of view that trust cannot be eliminated from human relationships, least of all relationships with professionals. Given this fact, an ethic based on mistrust and suspicion must, by the nature of human relationships, ultimately fail. To be sure, living wills, contracts if one wants them, durable powers of attorney, or appointment of a patient advocate or health care manager can diminish some of the vulnerability of trust relationships. In the end, however, all of these arrangements attempt to displace trust to some degree from the physician or professional and locate it elsewhere—but trust still remains as guarantor of the deed itself.

Given the empirical inevitability of trust in professional relationships, what is needed are not attempts to eradicate it, but rather a reconstruction of professional ethics grounded in the ineradicability of trust. Such an ethic of trust must be based on the "internal morality" of each profession,[13] those ethical obligations that arise from the nature of each profession, and the kind of human activity each profession encompasses.

The features of our trust relationships with professionals are, taken singly, not unique. What is specific to them is the peculiar constellation of urgency, intimacy, unavoidability, unpredictability, and extraordinary vulnerability within which trust must be given. It is this context that makes trusting professional relationships so problematic, so fragile, and so easily ruptured. A number of factors in contemporary society and medical practice have conspired to threaten and destroy this fragile fabric and to create a growing mistrust of trust that is damaging to patients as well as to professionals.

The Ethos and Ethics of Distrust

The Milieu of Medical Practice

Distrust of professionals, especially doctors and lawyers, is not a new phenomenon. Venal, greedy, incompetent, dishonest, and insensitive professionals have never been a rarity. They have been the satirist's favorites for a long time.[14]

Their acid comments have their origin in real experiences of the sick. In part, they arise from the gross misbehavior of professionals themselves and, in part, from the hostility of the sick to a fate that forces them to seek out physicians and then to pay for something they do not want in the first place. Because of our resentment at our loss of freedom, and at the powerlessness that serious illness imposes on all of us, the physician, good or bad, has always been a lightning rod for the frustrations of the sick.

In the last two or three decades, these perennial sources of distrust have been reinforced and expanded by a wide variety of events within and outside medicine— the malpractice crisis; the commercialization of medical care by advertising and entrepreneurialism; the excessive income and free-spending lifestyle of some physicians; the bottom-line, marketplace, "pay-before-we-treat" policies of hospitals and some doctors; the depersonalization of large group prepayment practices; physicians' growing preferences for 9 to 5 jobs and time off; the retreat from general to specialty practice; the early retirements. The list is long and growing daily.

As a result, patients, as the opinion polls show, increasingly think doctors are less available, less interested in them, and more interested in money than they used to be. In self-defense, patients feel they must take charge of their own care, do their own research about their symptoms and their doctors, and even order their own tests to become as informed as the doctor in order to be sure of getting good care. The doctor is, in this view, merely one resource among many.

The eroding effect of these attitudes on the trust relationship is clear. Wariness replaces trust. Physicians and patients approach each other as potential enemies rather than friends. Patients perceive doctors as less interested in them than in their money, more interested in time off than service, and more exploiters than stewards of medical knowledge. For many, the whole enterprise of medicine has increasingly called forth the principle of *caveat emptor* rather than the principles of fidelity to trust, beneficence, and effacement of self-interest.

These erosive tendencies within medicine have been reinforced by powerful forces within the social fabric of our times. Participatory democracy, better public education, the attention of the media, a mistrust of authority and of experts in general have all weakened the trust relationship. On the positive side, they encourage greater independence in patient decisions and thus help to neutralize the traditional paternalism of the professions. This is a salubrious move to more adult, open, and honest relationships. Indeed, the problem now is often the absolutization of autonomy, which must be tempered by the interests of third parties, and the moral right of physicians to refuse to do what they consider to be unethical. The line between healthy protection of patients' autonomy and dangerous depreciation of medical expertise is becoming more difficult to define.

The Ethics of Distrust

The most serious outcome of the erosion of trust is the emergence of an ethics of distrust. The formal and ultimately most destructive attack is on the very concept and possibility of trust relationships with professionals. Perhaps most serious of all, an ethics of distrust compromises the chance of achieving the purposes of professional relationships. Can a sick person be healed—made whole again—when he is suspicious of the motives and methods of his healer? A sick person must be empowered to heal himself. Is this possible when the person empowering is suspected of fostering her own self-interest? Can a client feel that her just cause is safe in the hands of a venal lawyer? Can a parishioner be served or reconciled with God if she cannot see the minister as a reliable avenue of access to spiritual healing? Not only is trust totally ineradicable from professional relationships, but the cultivation of trust is indispensable to the *telos* of each profession.

An ethos of distrust asserts the radical impossibility of trust in professional relationships.[15] Using medicine as an example, the ethics of distrust asserts that physicians cannot know all of a patient's values, that medicine deals only with a subset of things important to human fulfillment, and that physicians, by the very nature of their profession, necessarily place medical values over all other values. Moreover, since physicians are human, they have personal values that they cannot suppress. Physicians, therefore, select and weight the facts to be presented on the basis of their own rather than the patient's perceptions of what is good. Even so-called medical facts are tinged with value desiderata to such a degree that there are no value-free facts. Finally, we cannot trust in some standard of virtues inherent in professional practices that will protect the patient against the doctor's value system. The virtues of a profession are not intrinsic to that profession but are derivative from a wide variety of ethical and philosophical systems. There is nothing in the nature of medicine, law, or ministry *per se* that entails honesty, compassion, fidelity to trust, or suppression of self-interest; the so-called internal morality of the professions is a fiction. In this view, an ethos of distrust assumes the formal character of an ethics of distrust.

An ethics of distrust entails that professionals and those who seek their help assume primarily a self-protective stance. Patients must seek strict contractual relationships with their doctors. Specific instructions as to care must be spelled out by patients and must be observed to the letter by physicians. In addition, for further protection, some patients insist on the interjection of a presumably objective third party who will be the patient's advocate in place of the physician (or other professional) and who will monitor the physician's compliance with the terms of the contract.

There are empirical and conceptual difficulties in such an ethos and ethics of distrust. The empirical ineradicability of trust has already been discussed. Mechanisms proposed to bypass this ineradicability are illusory. If, for example, we prefer an ombudsman or health care manager to help us make decisions, we merely displace our trust from the physician to some other person. This person is still able to interject his or her own values into clinical decisions. The manager is susceptible to being coopted by the physician, the family, societal expectations, or self-interest. Doubtless, in some cases, patients would be better served by an ombudsman than by the professional. But this is by no means assured in the majority of cases. It introduces a serious and dangerous impediment to the discretionary latitude essential in professional decisions and action. The possibilities of confusion and conflict of opinion are multiplied. The patient will still have to trust one of the parties in any dispute between professionals and lay advocates. What is best is a decision with both technical and moral components.

The ethos and ethics of distrust confer a legalistic quality on relationships with professionals—one that leads to ethical minimalism. Professionals will tend to limit themselves to the precise letter of agreement. They will feel free of the expectation that they are advocates, counselors, and protectors of the patient's welfare. The professional's necessity to efface self-interest will be blunted, since legalistic and contractual relationships call upon the participants to protect their own self-interest, not that of the other party—except to the extent the contract requires. The impetus to do the extra work that requires some compromise of self-interest is blunted, if not destroyed entirely. These attitudes are already evident in professional relationships. They will be legitimated and reinforced by an ethos based in mistrust.

In addition to its empirical impossibility, there are conceptual and logical difficulties in a radical ethos of distrust. The fact that some physicians have violated their trust relationship does not vitiate the concept of trust. Other physicians do in fact respect it. Moreover, the fact that trust cannot be guaranteed, or may be respected only in part, cannot eradicate its reality in human and professional relationships.

It is true also that all of a patient's good is not subsumed in her medical good. Indeed, we have argued elsewhere that medical good is only one of the components of the complex notion of patient good, and that the key concept is beneficence in trust.[16] The doctor has an obligation to help define the patient's medical good, that is, the good that the recommended treatment can achieve. In this the physician is, or should be, the expert. But if the physician is to heal in any true sense, he must place the medical good in the context of the patient's assessment of his total good. In this the patient is the expert. The whole concept of patient autonomy is vitiated if it is assumed that trust entails granting to the physician determination of the other levels of good beyond medical good. The other levels of the patient's good include the patient's own assessment of what is good given his values, age, sex, occupation, aspirations, and the myriad things each of us as individuals may think more important than medical good or that would modify the degree and kind of medical treatment we would choose.

The logic of the argument against trust fails because its target is a gratuitous concept of global trust. This is not what the concept of trust in professionals need entail. We trust professionals in realms in which they have expertise. We trust them not to use that expertise to exploit our vulnerability for their own interests. We trust them for accurate information, and we trust them to empower and enable us to place their recommendations into the full context of our own hierarchy of values. We also trust them to carry out the procedures in which they are skilled and that we cannot perform for ourselves.

But, it will be argued, even in the presentation of the medical facts and indications, trust is an incoherent concept because facts and values are never separable; the physician's personal and professional values cannot help but color the way he presents his data. This is not the place to deal with such a fundamental epistemological problem as the fact–value dichotomy. However, it is worthwhile to consider some examples in which it seems clear that, in a real sense, fact and value are separable.

If a child falls out of a tree, fact and value decisions have to be made by parents and physician. Whether or not the skull is fractured, the spleen is ruptured, or shock is present, are all fact questions. Physical examination and X-rays will establish the kind and degree of fracture and provide a basis for what needs to be done mechanically to set it right. The choice of mechanical procedures is based on empirical facts related to risk, effectiveness in healing, restoring function, and the like. Personal values cannot change the physical signs or X-ray images.

Values enter the process when the factual data are used as a basis for choice between alternative treatments. Assuming that the child cannot make her own decision for reasons of incompetence, parents will weigh the alternative choices presented to them—treatment or no treatment, types of fracture reduction or anesthesia, functional result expected, length of rehabilitation period, pain, and dozens of other factors that go into an assessment of what is good for this child.

At this point, the process becomes a dialogue and a dialectic between fact and value. In this dialogue the doctor cannot be expected to know what is best for the totality of the child's well-being, but he is expert in what is medically wrong, what can be done, what can be expected, and what alternatives are available if healing or cure is to occur. To trust the doctor does not mean that we expect him to know everything important to the child and her parents. Rather, they must trust him to enable and empower them to make their own choice based on the most reliable facts.

The physician, of course, can shape the decision by the way he presents the factual data. He may give a higher value to health and medical care than the patient because of his professional commitment. He may also interject his own values or prejudices about life, politics, religion, and so on into the dialogue, either openly or covertly. The fact that this may happen does not mean that it must happen or that it is impossible to dissociate personal and professional values from medical indications. The fact is that some, indeed many, physicians are sensitive to their power to shape decisions covertly or overtly. While trust cannot be absolute or cover every aspect of the relationship with professionals, professionals can and do dissociate their personal and professional values, to varying degrees, from their recommendations.

That this dissociation is not perfect is not surprising given that professional relationships are, and will remain, relationships between humans. The absence of perfection does not make the concept invalid. It only underscores the need for a clarification of the content and the extent of trust in professional relationships. A refurbished ethic of trust will accept the fact that trust cannot be absolute, that it can be and is violated, but that nonetheless its ineradicability makes fidelity to trust a central obligation in all professional relationships.

The Ethics of Trust Restructured

Trust in professionals can no longer be absolute or open-ended, much as physicians and even some patients might wish it to be. Public education about medicine and medical ethics, the prominence of patient autonomy as a central principle of professional ethics, and the potential conflict between the physician's and patient's best interest all necessitate a more restricted and realistic view. Nevertheless, the ineradicability of trust mandates that it remain a central element in any coherent ethic of the professions.

Since trust is a permanent feature of human relating, fidelity to trust is an indispensable virtue of the good professional—lawyer, doctor, chaplain, or teacher. Without this virtue, the relationship with a professional cannot attain its end. It becomes a lie and a means of exploitation of vulnerability rather than a means of helping and healing. If there is any meaning to professional ethics, it must revolve around the obligation of **fidelity to trust**.

But what is to be entrusted to the professional? Clearly, from what has been said, patients should not entrust to the physician the responsibility for determining the totality of their good. Only the patient or the morally valid surrogate can know this. Physicians must not assume that they are entrusted with such a broad mandate. Some patients may feel overwhelmed by having to make a choice. Some may not trust anyone but the physician. Then, they might ask the physician what she thinks is best. Patients should be encouraged and enabled to make their own decisions. But if the patient empowers her to make the decision, the physician cannot refuse to help. That would constitute moral abandonment. Under these circumstances, the physician must make every effort to learn as much as she can about the many dimensions of what constitutes the patient's best interests. Then, under these unusual circumstances, the physician must be particularly self-critical. She should attempt to place the medical good within the larger context of the patient's total good, his value system, way of life, life history, spiritual and temporal commitments, and so on, as precisely as possible. The temptation to overstep the authority even when the patient provides the mandate must be resisted.

In an ethic of trust, the physician is impelled to develop a relationship with the patient from the very outset that includes becoming familiar with who and what the patient is and how she wants to meet the serious challenges of illness, disability, and death. It is essential that the physician help the patient to anticipate certain critical decisions, like withholding or withdrawing life-sustaining treatments, cardiopulmonary resuscitation, request for assisted death, abortion, and the like. The physician must prepare the patient for these eventualities before they become urgent or the patient loses competence. Patients should be able to rely on the physician for the proper timing, sensitivity, and degree of detail appropriate in each case. These cannot be written into a contract. They must be entrusted to the physician or a physician substitute.

In an ethic of trust, the physician is obliged to present clinical data as free as possible of personal or professional bias. Fidelity to trust precludes manipulation, coercion, or deception in obtaining consent. It requires assisting patients to perform the calculus of effectiveness, benefit, and burden as carefully as the situation permits. It is here that other virtues intersect, virtues such as intellectual honesty and humility. What is known must be distinguished from what is uncertain or simply unknown. The indispensability of keeping information up-to-date is obvious. Consultation with, or reference to, those with more experience or skill, or with closer congruence with the patient's values, is required. When the patient's and physician's values are sharply at variance, the physician should decline to enter the relationship or withdraw from it graciously, with candor, and without recrimination.

A realistic ethic of trust does not absolutize the professional's fiduciary role. Nor does it ignore the realities that may compromise trust, like those enumerated by Veatch—for example, the potential intrusion of the physician's personal and professional values, the complexity of the notion of the patient's best interests, and the difficulty of disassociating fact and value.

Nor does an ethic of trust ignore the sad facts of incompetence, quackery, fraud, inadequate self-regulation and peer review of the addicted or alcoholic professional. To recognize the ineradicability of trust is not, therefore, to argue against regulation of the professional by licensure, educational and certification procedures, quality controls, periodic relicensure, and liability laws. Professionals are ordinary humans called by the nature of the activities in which they engage to extraordinary degrees of obligation and trust. Living wills, durable power of attorney, and inquires into competence are all legitimate measures that those who seek professional help are entitled to invoke. A certain degree of distrust based on experience of the caprices of human behavior is unavoidable.

But these reasonable constraints on trust do not justify an ethic of distrust that takes fidelity to trust relationships to be invalid and impossible. That trust may be violated in varying degrees does not entail the inevitability of its violation. Moreover, even if all the current measures that place restraint on trust were implemented, an ineradicable residuum of trust would remain. It is with the acknowledgment of this residuum, its enhancement and strengthening, that an ethic of trust is most concerned. A restructured ethic of trust therefore recognizes simultaneously the origins of distrust and the ineradicability of trust.

On balance, an ethic of trust is more realistic, conceptually sounder, and phenomenologically more consistent than an ethic of distrust. To highlight trust in professional relationships, to make it explicit and more precise, is to provide the very protection an ethic of distrust seeks but cannot reach. Older notions of absolute trust are inadequate and were always so. What is needed is a redefinition of trust relationships consistent with the contemporary context of autonomy, participatory democracy, and the moral pluralism of the interacting parties in professional relationships.

Clearly, an ethic of trust must go beyond principle- and duty-based ethics to an ethics of virtue and character. This is consistent with the current revival of interest in virtue theories. In general and professional ethics, it also calls for a reconciliation between autonomy and beneficence along lines we have detailed elsewhere as beneficence in trust. More attention to character formation and professionalization is essential, since virtue is best taught by practice in the presence of teachers who themselves are models of virtuous behavior.[17,18]

It goes without saying that trust must be earned and merited by performance and fidelity to its implications. Professionals cannot expect to be trusted simply because they are professionals. The ineradicability of trust is a source of obligations, not of privilege. Professionals who resent the queries and the skepticism of their patients or clients are insensitive to the changed climate of professional relationships. They fail to sense the predicament of vulnerability in which those who seek their help must find themselves.

Essential to an ethics of trust is the professional's realization that if there is distrust, the problem may not rest entirely with the patient or client. Trust is easily destroyed, sometimes over minor failures—forgetting to provide results of a test, failing to perform some needed service, or sidestepping some important question. Trust must be engendered and built up gradually by fidelity to promise from the very first moments of a professional relationship. It is as fragile a phenomenon as it is an ineradicable dimension of a helping and healing relationship.

Difficult as these requirements may be, the effort to meet them is worthwhile. The alternative is an ethic based on the presumption of distrust, which can only degenerate into a minimalistic and legalistic ethic that is no ethic at all but merely a relationship of mutual self defense. Professionals no longer under any obligation of fidelity will feel free to pursue self-interest. Patients or clients will harbor the illusion that they can protect themselves from all harm by regulation and personal management of every potential risk. Such a scenario will not only destroy any concept of professional responsibility but will be far more perilous than a strengthened and restructured ethic of trust.

Notes

1. Robert M. Veatch, "Is Trust of Professionals a Coherent Concept?", *Ethics, Trust, and the Professions: Philosophical and Cultural Aspects* ed. Edmund D. Pellegrino, Robert

M. Veatch, and John P. Langan, (Washington, DC: Georgetown University Press, 1991), pp. 159–176.

2. Bernard Barber, *The Logic and Limits of Trust* (New Brunswick, NJ: Rutgers University Press, 1983), p. 9.

3. Ibid., p. 135.

4. Niklas Luhmann, *Trust and Power,* ed. T. Burns and P. Gianfranco (Ann Arbor, MI: Books on Demand, 1979), p. 30.

5. Ibid., p. 39.

6. Annette Baier, "Trust and Anti-Trust," *Ethics* 96(2) (January 1986):231–260. Quote from p. 259.

7. Barber, *Logic and Limits,* pp. 14–16.

8. Baier, "Trust and Anti-Trust," p. 245.

9. Edmund D. Pellegrino, "Character, Virtue and Self-Interest in the Ethics of the Professions," *The Journal of Contemporary Health Law and Policy* 5 (Spring 1989):53–73.

10. Edmund D. Pellegrino, "Rationing Health Care: The Ethics of Medical Gatekeeping," *The Journal of Contemporary Health Law and Policy* 2 (1986):23–45.

11. William F. May, *The Physician's Covenant* (Philadelphia: Westminster Press, 1983).

12. David C. Thomasma, "The Ethics of Caring for Vulnerable Individuals," *Reflection on Ethics* (Washington, DC.: American Speech-Language-Hearing Association, 1990), pp. 39–45.

13. Edmund D. Pellegrino, "The Healing Relationship: The Architectonics of Clinical Medicine," *The Clinical Encounter,* ed. E. Shelp (Dordrecht, Holland: D. Reidel, 1983), pp. 153–178.

14. Mary B. Mahowald, "The Physician," *The Power of the Professions,* ed. R. W. Clarke and R. O. Lawry (Lanham, MD: University Press of America, 1988), pp. 119–131.

15. Allen Buchanan, "The Physician's Knowledge and the Patient's Best Interest," *Ethics, Trust, and the Professions,* ed. Pellegrino, Veatch, and Langan, pp. 93–112; Dan W. Brock, "Facts and Values in the Physician–Patient Relationship," ibid., pp. 113–138; and Robert M. Veatch, "Is Trust . . . Coherent?", pp. 159–173.

16. Edmund D. Pellegrino and David C. Thomasma, *For the Patient's Good: The Restoration of Beneficence in Health Care* (New York: Oxford University Press, 1988).

17. Charles S. Bosk, *Forgive and Remember: Managing Medical Failure* (Chicago: University of Chicago Press, 1979).

18. George Agich, "Professionalism and Ethics of Health Care," *The Journal of Medicine and Philosophy* 5(3) (September 1980):187–199.

6

Compassion

If there is one criticism of medicine and physicians that is widespread among patients today and painful for physicians to hear, it is a perceived deficiency in compassion. This criticism is usually accompanied by a plea for physicians, nurses, all health professionals, and health care institutions to couple their use of medical knowledge and skill with a better perception of the predicament of illness in the persons they are attending. This call for compassion goes directly to the central concern of this book: the character of the physician. Compassion cannot be expressed neatly in a principle, rule, guideline, or description of a duty. It summates the whole of the character, virtues, and vices of physicians and nurses. Its components are many—psychological, sociological, cultural, ethnic, and intellectual. But compassion is also a moral virtue in the classical sense in which we are using the term in this book—a habitual disposition, to act in a certain way, a way that facilitates and enriches the *telos* or purpose of whatever human acts we perform. In medicine, of course, the act in question is the act of healing, helping, and caring for someone who is ill. Compassion is the character trait that shapes the cognitive aspect of healing to fit the unique predicament of *this* patient.

In this chapter, we will focus on the philosophical aspects of compassion—its nature, its components, and its expression in the medical relationship. We recognize that compassion closely parallels the theological virtue of charity, but it is not entirely congruent with it.

The Virtue of Compassion

Compassion is an essential virtue of medical practice. A good physician does not just apply cognitive data from the medical literature to the particular patient by reason of a catalog or "cook-book" of indications. Rather, the good physician cosuffers with the patient. A bond is created by which the data are filtered into the particular circumstances of the patient. The pristine etymology of words, especially those imported into a language to enrich its indigenous vocabulary, is often a guide to the emotion or idea the word is intended to encompass. Nowhere is this clearer than in the derivation of compassion from the Latin words—*com* (together) and *pati* (to suffer)—or, as the *Oxford English Dictionary* puts it, "suffering together with another, participation in suffering, fellow-feeling."[1] Compassion suggests strongly the ideas of cosuffering, of fellowship in the experience, of comprehension of "what it's like," and even of taking upon oneself something of another's pain and making it, to the extent possible, one's own. To be compassionate is to be disposed to see, as well as feel, what a trial, tribulation, or illness has wrought in the life of this person's here-and-now suffering. Compassion is not measurable by the psychological testing of a physician or nurse. It is truly a cosuffering. Compassion is embedded in a personal dynamic relationship. It is definable in terms of the interaction of two persons, not solely of one or the other. The existence of compassion, on the other hand, can only be attested to by the person who is suffering and in an actual relationship with a *particular* physician or nurse.

Compassion is a compound of affect, attitude, word, gesture, and language, but compassion is also a virtue in the classical sense. This means that it encompasses a moral and an intellectual component. Compassion, like other virtues, is related to emotional states out of which it may emerge and with which it may be expressed. But virtues are also more than emotions, and it is this extra dimension that is most significant for our discussion of compassion as a virtue.

The Moral Aspect of Compassion

Let us look at the moral component—at why compassion is a necessary, habitual attribute of the morally authentic healer. If virtues are dispositions to act in ways that most effectively advance attainment of the end of a human activity, then compassion is a moral virtue of medicine and all healing. This is so because the physician or nurse cannot "heal," that is, make whole again, without feeling and knowing the nuances of a particular patient's predicament of illness. The physician cannot heal if, in the act of healing (or attempted healing), the healer violates some value or feeling of the person to be healed or shows disrespect, lack of concern, indifference, or disengagement from this person's way of seeing her predicament. We cannot restore whatever measure of healthful harmony may be possible to the functioning of body and mind if we create an element of disharmony through the healing relationship itself.

Moreover, to introduce such disharmony, not to guard against it, or to justify it out of expediency is to violate the covenant of trust with the patient, namely, that we will use our medical knowledge in the patient's interest. Since the virtue of compassion is indispensable to attaining the end of medicine, its presence or absence in the healer is a matter of moral concern.

The Intellectual Aspect of Compassion

In addition to the moral dimension, there is an intellectual component to the virtue of compassion. It consists in the disposition habitually to comprehend, assess, and weigh the uniqueness of this patient's predicament of illness. Here, again, it is the end that shapes the virtue. That end is healing, helping, and curing. That end may be served in many ways, since it is defined in terms of the patient's good, which consists not only of the medical good, but also the good as the patient perceives it herself, or her good as a human person or spiritual being.

The strictly medical good must be shaped to fit this person's unique circumstances, her life story, aspirations, hopes, failures, fears, sentiments, and so on at the moment in which the decision is to be made and in conformity with how these are perceived by the patient for the future. Compassion, in this sense, consists of assisting the patient to balance her assessment of what is good with the good that medicine can offer. This requires a certain discernment of what in fact, is the patient's predicament. In this, the physician must discern from his own affective responses of empathy, sympathy, and even pity those elements that genuinely reflect the patient's predicament.

To carry out this cognitive function of the virtue of compassion requires, paradoxically, a certain *epoché,* a suspending of the attachment that the affective component requires, so that we may objectively stand back and measure, weight, feel, test, question—in short, uses the tools of medical diagnosis to define the predicament and to symbolize it in appropriate language. The physician's effort should be to shape treatment recommendations to accommodate all those things—personal, emotional, and social, as well as physical—that make *this* illness a unique experience for *this* person.

Compassion, thus, has an objective component that can be ascertained by the methods of medicine and grasped cognitively and that, together with the moral component, makes it a virtue. As a virtue, compassion also strives for a mean. If the physician identifies too closely as cosufferer with the patient, she loses the objectivity essential to the most precise assessment of what is wrong, of what can be done, and of what should be done to meet those needs. Excessive cosuffering also impedes and may even paralyze the physician in a state of inaction. Cosuffering also has the danger of so close an identification with the patient's suffering that the physician unconsciously imposes her values on the patient. To identify too closely is to do what the physician might want done in similar circumstances. This is a species of paternalism even though it may be the result of empathy and sympathy.

Four Elements of Compassion

There must be a proper balance between compassion as a virtue, its component parts, and other virtues of medicine, particularly competence. The latter virtue demands accurate assessment of the clinical evidence, clarity of reasoning, and judiciousness of judgment. The monitoring and modulating virtue here, as with the relationship between all the virtues, is prudence.

Compassion should be distinguished from empathy, mercy, and pity, with which it is closely associated and with which it may be confused. These three affective states also dispose to a certain identity with the patient's plight, but not in precisely the same way that compassion does.

Mercy involves "compassion shown to one who is in one's power and has no claim on kindness."[2] Mercy thus has the connotations of forbearance or charity shown by someone superior to someone inferior. As Portia says in the famous speech, "mercy seasons justice," so that "earthly power doth them show like God's."[3] Thus, there is in mercy the idea of leniency, of not applying strict justice. Compassion is a necessary element of mercy—feeling something of a person's predicament before showing leniency.

But there is no place for mercy in this sense in the medical relationship. To be sure, there is a sense in which the patient is in the doctor's power. But it is this fact, plus the doctor's promise to help, that makes compassion a moral obligation. The patient does indeed have a claim on the doctor's compassion, but she is not an inferior, but vulnerable fellow human being to whom the doctor is bound to help by the covenant of trust.

Empathy is another related affective state, that is, a capacity to imagine oneself as another, or to project one's personality into another's life sufficiently to feel and understand the other person's feelings. Empathy is broader than compassion, which focuses on one specific aspect of another's experience, that is, his suffering. An actor may be empathetic with the character he is portraying and share many of the character's ideas, thoughts, or actions, yet not necessarily share the suffering. Empathy enables one to enter the emotional world of the other person. This is the first step toward compassion, but it is not synonymous with it.

Sympathy is closer to compassion because it is concerned with sharing of feelings and a sense of fellowship with other humans, regardless of whether they are in adversity. Sympathy has broad psychological, social, ethical, and cultural aspects. It may or may not lead to sharing of suffering or to a compulsion to help another. Sympathy lacks the specificity of compassion, although it may embrace it under a broader umbrella of shared human fellowship.

Finally, there is pity, which is furthest from the sense of compassion, which we take to be a necessary virtue. Pity has unfortunate historical connotations of condescension, a feeling for the lowly conditions of others who are unfortunate or not one's equals. Pity also had the connotation described above for mercy, forbearance for an inferior being. Pity has the same limitation in the medical relationship as mercy, since it is based on a notion of inequality. The inequality in the medical relationship is not one of intrinsic inequality or the person. It is a consequence of the wounded humanity of the person who is ill. It is not an act of pity, but of a moral obligation to help or heal the sick.

Compassion and Friendship

Compassion therefore is a virtue distinct from mercy, pity, empathy, or sympathy, though these affective states may be more or less closely related. Compassion focuses on coexperiencing another's suffering. Compassion includes an ability to objectify what another person is feeling in symbolic form, that is, in our speech, our body language, and our participation in the "story" of the other's illness. This is the way that a friend who helps us live through and talk through the experiences of illness, sorrow, hospital admission, loss, or grief makes his compassion evident to us. When a physician acts similarly in her relationship with the patient, she cosuffers as a friend cosuffers.

But the physician brings something the friend usually lacks—a technical and scientific component that places the patient's story within a paradigmatic context of others with the same symptoms, signs, or disease. In a medical context, this technical component is not a foreign element or a contradiction of compassion. The compassionate physician is not the one who demeans or neglects the objective, technical, or scientific data. Nothing is more inconsistent with compassion than the well-meaning, empathetic, but incompetent clinician. Competence must coexist with compassion. It is only when the physician uses technical information, without reference to the things that make *this* experience unique for *this* patient, that she can be noncompassionate.

At times, technical competence must be predominant—that is, when the patient is under anesthesia and the surgeon is anastomosing coronary vessels. But preoperatively and postoperatively, the personal and emotional sharing of the experience takes precedence. At every point in a medical relationship, compassion and competence go hand in hand as necessary and mutually reinforcing virtues essential to attainment of the ends and purposes of the clinical encounter.

Conclusion

Virtues like compassion and integrity are even more readily seen to be related to all the other virtues, like justice or fortitude or temperance. This is because, in discussing a virtue, one must consider many different components that directly relate to other virtues. In our discussion of compassion, for example, we also considered empathy, sympathy, mercy, pity, and friendship, as well as, peripherally, *agape* and justice. These relationships underscore the fact that medicine itself is a virtue when it is practiced in conjunction with patients. Both the patient and the physician develop these virtues, which are part of the larger process of healing.

Notes

1. "Compassion," *Oxford English Dictionary* (Oxford: Clarendon Press, 1961), vol. 2, p. 714.
2. "Mercy," *Oxford English Dictionary* (Oxford: Clarendon Press, 1961), vol. 6, pp. 351–352.
3. William Shakespeare, *The Merchant of Venice*, A.IV, S.I, 11s. 163ff.

7

Phronesis:
Medicine's Indispensable Virtue

Few words are as easily misconstrued as prudence. In its contemporary usage, it suggests timidity, undue concern for self-interest, unwillingness to take risks, a narrow pragmatism, and a range of other, less than admirable traits. Yet, in the ancient and medieval worlds, prudence was the capstone virtue, the link between the intellectual and the moral life. In this chapter, we argue that prudence, properly construed, is an indispensable virtue of the medical life, essential to the *telos* of medicine—a right and good healing action for a particular patient—and essential as well to the *telos* of the physician *qua* human being, the life of fulfillment and flourishing.

Phronesis is the term Aristotle used for the virtue of practical wisdom, the capacity for moral insight, the capacity, in a given set of circumstances, to discern what moral choice or course of action is most conducive to the good of the agent or the activity in which the agent is engaged. *Phronesis* is the intellectual virtue that disposes us habitually to attain truth for the sake of action, as opposed to truth for its own sake, which is speculative wisdom or *sophia*.

Phronesis occupies a special place among the virtues as the link between the intellectual virtues—those that dispose to truth (science, art, intuitive and theoretical wisdom, etc.)—and those that dispose to good character (temperance, courage, justice, generosity, etc.). *Phronesis* tells us when the end or the good to which we are tending as persons or as carpenters, doctors, and so on is in jeopardy. *Phronesis* provides a grasp of the end, of the good, for the agent and the work in which he or she is engaged. Prudence enables us to discern which means are most appropriate to the good in particular circumstances.

This concept of practical wisdom prevailed in Western moral philosophy relatively unchanged until the thirteenth century, when it was enriched and expanded by Thomas Aquinas. Aquinas used the term "prudence," subsuming Aristotle's meanings of *phronimos* and enriching it with the insights he gleaned from Revelation. Prudence was not the sickly concept it has become for many people in the contemporary world. Rather, for Aquinas and much of the medieval and post-medieval world, prudence was the capstone virtue, the link between the intellectual, moral, and supernatural virtues. It was the indispensable connection between cognition of the good and the disposition to seek it in particular acts.

Prudence, thus, takes into account the full breadth of Aristotelian *phronesis*, but in addition, its discerning capacity extends to the supernatural virtues of faith, hope, and charity—as well as to the moral and intellectual virtues recognized by Aristotle. For Aquinas, prudence was a *recta ratio agibilium,* a right way of acting. It was contrasted with speculative knowledge, *recta ratio speculabilium,* and art, *recta ratio factibilium.*

Prudence is a guide to the right way of acting with respect to all the virtues. It provides the capacity or disposition to select the right means and the right balance between means and good ends. It orients us to moral truth, to the moral quality of particular acts and their relationship to the ends of human nature. Prudence itself is shaped by the universal moral guideline that we must seek good and avoid evil. Prudence helps us to discern, at this moment, in this situation, what action, given the uncertainties of human cognition, will most closely approximate the right and the good. Like *phronesis,* prudence rests on reason, but it adds the notion of appreciation of the realities of a faith commitment that did not exist for Aristotle. Prudence, as well as the other virtues, enables individuals to recognize their place in history and in context, and how the moral life needs completion and fulfillment in the relation of all the virtues to one another.[1]

Prudence shapes the other virtues, since it relates all the means at our disposal to attain the good specific to us as humans or to the work in which we are engaged. The other virtues—justice, courage, moderation, and others—are dispositions that must be instantiated in a certain way in particular concrete acts. The proper instantiation of each virtue is guided by prudence in particular practical moral choices.

Prudence does not guarantee certitude. It recognizes the anxiety of choice in complex circumstances. It does enable us to assess the complexities as accurately as possible and to approximate, as closely as the circumstances permit, what would be right and good, and what would not jeopardize the good or frustrate the virtues. Prudence is not synonymous with the practice of casuistry. Josef Pieper, one of the most astute commentators on the virtues, warns against that error by pointing out that casuistry is a method. When well done, casuistry depends upon the proper use of prudence, but it is not prudence itself, since prudence is a virtue and casuistry a method.[2] Unless the casuist is endowed with the virtue of prudence, the result of his or her casuistic analysis may be seriously in error. We shall return to this point below in our discussion of the place of prudence in medicine.

Prudence in Medicine

In his definition of virtue, Aristotle focuses on two things: the good for human beings and the good for the work we do: "The excellence of human beings will also be the state of character which makes a person good and which makes that person do his or her work well."[3] In this book we will address only one of these two definitions of virtue: the excellence that makes a person do his or her work well.

It is far beyond the scope of this work to attempt to define those excellences that might make a person *qua* person good. Such a definition requires agreement on what it is to be human, on what the proper goal and purpose of life is or should be, and a clear relationship between the right and the good. In our morally pluralistic society, those are matters of vigorous debate and the widest divergence of opinion. Indeed, it is lack of agreement on those questions that stands in the way of any general theory of virtue despite the recent renewal of interest in virtue among ethicists.

The matter is somewhat simpler when we concentrate on the second part of Aristotle's definition, on the work to be done—in this case, on medicine as a certain kind of human activity. We can define, with some hope of agreement, what the ends of medicine are. The ultimate end is the health of individuals and society, while the more proximate end is a right and good healing action for a specific patient.[4] These ends constitute the good of medicine, that to which the virtues of the physician *qua* physician should be directed.

We have examined the ends of medicine in Chapter 4. Let us look in more detail here at the proximate end of medicine as it is exemplified in the clinical encounter between a sick person needing and seeking health and a physician who offers to provide that help. A right and good healing action is the aim of both the doctor and the patient. The right of correct action is what is scientifically and technically appropriate. But the action also must be morally good, that is, it should be in the interests of the patient. "Interests" include not only the medical good, that which medical knowledge dictates, but also the good as interpreted by the patient in terms of his own values, lifestyle, aspirations, religious beliefs, and so on. A healing decision or action focuses on restoring the patient to at least the state he enjoyed before becoming ill, or to a state of higher satisfaction and health than had been reached previously, if at all possible. "Healing" is used here in its broadest sense. Even when it is not possible to cure or contain the disease, healing can occur if the patient is assisted to cope with her illness, is cared for as a continuing member of the human community, and is helped to confront dying and death when they are inevitable.

If these ends of medicine are to be attained, certain character traits are required of the physician, like compassion, fidelity to trust, honesty, intellectual humility, benevolence, and courage. These are, to use Aristotle's term, the "excellences" or virtues that enable the physician to do the work of medicine well. Among these virtues, prudence plays a special role because of the nature of medicine as an activity. Medicine, or more properly healing, is a practical enterprise requiring a fusion of technical competence and moral judgment.

Clinical judgment is essentially an exercise of prudence, the "right way of acting," to use Aquinas' definition of prudence, in a complex situation fraught with uncertainties. It is here that the clinician must discern what means are most appropriate to the ends, how to balance the benefits and harms in clinical interventions, and how to put the moral and technical issues in a proper relationship with each other.

If compassion, fidelity to trust, intellectual humility, and the other virtues intrinsic to healing are to be properly employed, there is need of prudence to guide them. Thus, in medical as in moral choice, prudence is the capstone or guiding virtue that influences the way the other virtues are exhibited in any given clinical situation. Prudence is therefore both an intellectual and a moral virtue in medicine, as it is in moral encounters generally.

Aristotle refers frequently to the *phronimos,* the person endowed with the virtue of *phronesis,* the individual of practical wisdom. Aristotle defines the virtuous action as one that the person of practical wisdom would decide. Let us examine a few examples of how the virtue of prudence might shape moral choice in the clinical context by its deployment of the virtues or the principles of medical ethics.

Prudence in the Clinical Context

Compassion surely is a virtue that the healing end of medicine entails. It consists of the capacity to share in the experience of illness, in the suffering of the patient. Compassion, like many virtues, aims toward a mean. If the physician is too compassionate and comes too close to the experience of suffering, he will lose the objectivity necessary for proper diagnosis and selection of treatment, thus defeating the end of medicine in its healing function. On the other hand, not to have compassion is to treat the patient as an object, as simply a particular instance of a disease process. The patient is divested of the rich particulars of age, occupation, sex, race, situation in life, values—all those particulars that define us as persons and give us identity.

There is no formula or calculus by which the physician can determine with accuracy at what point to strike the balance between compassion and objectivity, both of which are intrinsic to the healing end of medicine. It is here precisely that the virtue of prudence enters, enabling the physician to assess the relative weight of the means at her disposal, the therapeutic possibilities and outcomes and side effects, and the values and life circumstances of the patient, as well as his preferences and other factors. The point of balance is never the same for any series of patients. Prudence is necessary if the extremes of compassion or objectivity are not to neutralize each other.

Similar dilemmas occur with the virtue of honesty. In this era of autonomy and informed consent, patients are owed disclosure of the nature of their condition in sufficient detail to allow an informed choice among alternative modes of treatment. Deception, manipulation of consent, or selective presentation of data is, on the face of it, morally insupportable. Yet every clinician, and indeed any patient or family that has had the experience, knows that how the information is conveyed is of the utmost importance. Experienced clinicians moreover assert, with considerable accuracy, that they can get almost any decision they want, depending on how they use their authority and knowledge to present the choices.

On the other hand, to present too much, too soon, and before the gravity of the situation has been conveyed or the patient has accommodated to it, can be seriously harmful. If the benefits are presented too rosily, the patient's hopes may be unrealistically raised. If they are presented too starkly or bluntly, the patient may become so discouraged that she rejects a high risk or a temporarily painful but perhaps highly successful procedure. Again, we look to the physician's prudent judgment to mediate between presenting too much and too little information where there is no likelihood of a standardized approach.

When does obtaining consent become coercive? When should the physician try to persuade, and when is he unduly influencing the decision? Is it not tantamount to moral abandonment not to advise the patient on the basis of our best estimate of the interests of the patient? Yet if we express our own preferences, do we not subtly overmaster the vulnerable patient? The prudent physician is the one we expect to make these difficult distinctions on the basis of a character fixed in its disposition to act well, to keep the end of healing in its totality in view, and to modulate the application of means so as to foster but not frustrate that end.

Trust is an ineradicable element defining the morality of **the healing relationship**. Fidelity to trust is, therefore, a virtue entailed by that relationship. It is an essential disposition of the good physician or nurse, and its very ineradicability dictates that the violation of trust vitiates healing in any genuine sense.

Yet there are times when the healing end of medicine seems to tempt us, for what appear to be good reasons arising in the patient's interests, to broaden our understanding of trust in the patient's interests. What the physician means by trust and what the patient means may be quite different. Physicians want to be trusted to do the "right" thing, often meaning the medically right thing, that which satisfies the canons of good medicine. Can the physician, in an effort to help the patient, see the benefits of a particular treatment, engage the help of family or friends, soften the details of side effects, or minimize the patient's fears—all without the patient's knowledge? Is this a gross violation of trust or is it fidelity to the trust implicit in engaging a physician in the first place? The answer, in the abstract, might seem obvious, but buried in the context of a particular decision for a particular patient, it might well be another. In the concrete case, moral insight, or prudence as we have been describing it, is necessary if we are to do the morally best thing.

Similarly with **respect for persons**, surely the most important virtue in the healing relationship for many people. There is little doubt that the strong version of paternalism, which assumes that the patient can never know what is in his own interests, is not morally defensible.[5] But many ethicists would allow for weak paternalism, deciding for the patient, or even overriding her preferences when her competence is in doubt or variable.

Should a living will or durable power of attorney forbidding intubation be respected when the patient arrives in the emergency room cyanotic, acidotic, mentally confused, and struggling for breath? Should the patient with a severe burn or fresh spinal cord injury who expressed the desire to die shortly after arriving be healed? What about the young Christian Scientist with treatable meningococcus meningitis and meningococcemia, a temperature of 105°F, and mental confusion be allowed to refuse antibiotics? Regarding the patient with AIDS and probable central nervous system involvement, should her request for no treatment be respected?

What about the therapeutic privilege, a privilege we think should be used very infrequently, if at all? There are times when, if the evidence is unequivocal, disclosing the full nature of a disease or procedure will produce such deprivation of hope that patients will contemplate suicide, refuse lifesaving treatment, or request euthanasia, a new reality in the moral decision-making process. Does trust require the physician to disclose all the facts, independent of grave, discernible, probable harm to the patient? Or does the covenant of trust encompass the possibility of its violation to preserve another trust—to act in the immediate best interests of the patient as a person? What preserves personhood more safely—disclosure with loss of hope, alienation, and depression or the false hope born of withholding information?

In these and many other complex clinical decisions, the answers given in the abstract or as an exercise in balancing *prima facie* principles against one other might seem simpler than they are in practice. Here again we confront the need for moral insight, for that combination of intuitive grasp by natural inclination of what is right and good here, and how in this decision we call prudence to resolve these conflicts in ways no formula can guarantee. In the maelstrom of anxiety, uncertainty, and urgency characteristic of the medical encounter, it is the virtue of prudence to which we turn to tell us how to resolve our understanding of such virtues as honesty, fidelity to trust, respect for persons, and so on.

Such a conclusion is worrisome for those who see clinical decision making as an exercise in probability and stochastic reasoning or game theory. There is nothing intrinsically wrong with trying to make the process of moral choice as rigorous, explicit, and theoretically sound as possible, or even with constructing moral algorithms. What must be kept in mind, however, is that at every junction, some prudential assessment of competing values, principles, or virtues must be made. Without such decisions, the branching decision-making tree must stop growing. Like it or not, the decision analyst, as well as the clinician whose thought processes he wishes to describe, uses prudence. It is on the quality of that virtue that the ultimate moral quality of the decision depends.

There are other examples of virtues in medicine that need the mediation and ordering that prudence provides. Loyalty is another example. Loyalty is a disposition habitually to act right in relation to persons to whom we have special attachment— our families, patients, or professional colleagues. In actual practice, these attachments are overlapping and sometimes in serious conflict with each other. Our patients want and are owed a certain privilege to our availability and accessibility to our time. So do our families, to whom we have serious obligations. How do we divide our time, our emotional resources, and our presence among them? Who has first claim on our loyalty when we learn of a fellow physician's incompetence, substance abuse, or dishonesty?

A rule of principle-based analysis might give a "right" answer in general terms. But the actual decision is of necessity less clear-cut. Is it consistent with loyalty to the patient not to warn her against the less than competent surgeon, or the unscrupulous or money-minded colleague? When do we blow the whistle on the physician whose competence is compromised by substance abuse? The potential harms is these conflicts are not solved by yes–no bytes in a computer program. They present degrees of potential harm in human beings to whom we are attached, and not objects sandwiched against each other.

Prudence and Clinical Judgment

Is not what we have so laboriously tried to describe what clinicians have known for centuries as "clinical judgment"—a quasi-mystical intuitive grasp of the right thing to do? In some senses, if we eliminate the overtones of mysticism, we would agree, this is because, implicitly, clinical judgment requires the use of prudence. But to use prudence is not synonymous with prudence; a good clinical judgment is the end product of the use of prudence.

Let us elaborate a little further. Medical and clinical decisions generally require the closest integration of scientific and moral reasoning and judgment. One of the major achievements of contemporary biomedical ethics is to lay bare the moral roots of clinical decisions and to show how inextricably intertwined they are with the scientific and technical. Anyone who has had to unravel the intricacies of clinical choices in a concrete case knows that the decision is the product of an intimate dialogue between the clinical facts and the moral principles, values, or virtues.

Prudence is an essential element of the clinical judgment because prudence is, to repeat St. Aquinas' trenchant phrase *a recto ratio agibilium*—a right way of acting. In medicine this right way is to attain the healing purposes of medicine. To act in the patient's best interests, one needs both the intellectual virtues (theoretical wisdom, understanding and practical wisdom) and the moral virtues (generosity, self-control, etc.). Heretofore, clinical judgment put its emphasis on the use of prudence almost exclusively as ordering the intellectual virtues essential to good scientific decisions. Now we must be equally explicit about the moral judgment. Prudence, and *phronimos,* link the intellectual and moral virtues. This is precisely what is required for a good clinical judgment today. Hence prudence is the indispensable virtue for medicine. The practice of medicine is intellectual as well as moral, just as the virtues are.

Clearly, if virtue theory is to have a place in a comprehensive moral philosophy of medicine, its pivot must be the virtue of prudence or *phronesis.* Likewise, if general virtue theory is to be resuscitated, a fuller understanding of prudence is essential. It may be that prudence, besides linking the intellectual and moral virtues, may link the emotions with the virtues, perhaps closing the gap between cognition of the good and motivation to do the good. Prudence has this possibility, since it combines reason with disposition. But also, there is something "in virtue of which we stand well or badly with reference to the passions."[6] More than the other virtues, *phronesis* endows its possessor with the deliberative capacity to reason well with respect to the means to be used to attain the good of the activity in which we have been engaged.

Conclusion: The Good Person

For reasons stated earlier in this chapter, we have deliberately confined our discussion of the virtues to only one of the two aspects touched upon by Aristotle— that is, making us do the "work" (i.e., medicine) well. But virtues also are states of character that make a person good as a person as well. We prescinded the question of what constituted a good person in the more general sense. But we cannot escape the conclusion that a person who is a prudent physician cannot avoid being a good person in at least one sector of life. To pursue medicine virtuously is to move one toward happiness and fulfillment, albeit not the fullest expression of happiness. Prudence, habitually exhibited in medical practice, conduces to happiness, that is, to a satisfying life in medicine.

Notes

1. Alasdair C. MacIntyre, *Three Rival Versions of Moral Enquiry: Encyclopedia, Geneology, and Tradition* (Notre Dame, IN: Notre Dame University Press, 1990), p. 140.

2. Josef Pieper, *The Four Cardinal Virtues: Prudence, Justice, Fortitude, Temperance,* trans. Richard and Clara Winston et al. (New York: Harcourt, Brace & World, 1965).

3. Aristotle, *Nicomachean Ethics,* 1106, a22–24.

4. Edmund D. Pellegrino and David C. Thomasma, *A Philosophical Basis of Medical Practice: Toward a Philosophy and Ethic of the Healing Professions* (New York: Oxford University Press, 1981), pp. 119–152.

5. Edmund D. Pellegrino and David C. Thomasma, *For the Patient's Good: The Restoration of Beneficence in Health Care* (New York: Oxford University Press, 1989).

6. Aristotle, *Nicomachean Ethics,* 1105, b25–26.

8

Justice

Several years ago, medical ethics and the philosophy of medicine were little concerned with issues of cost containment and access to health care. Still less was there evidence of interest in theories of justice that might drive an equitable health delivery system. That situation has now changed. It has changed dramatically. Issues in economics and social justice have now come to predominate in medical ethics debates. Earlier, we asked if modern health care institutions can compete in today's marketplace and still maintain their fundamental commitments. At risk is the proper respect to be shown to each individual served by the institution. The same question holds for the health care provider. Under pressure to be an entrepreneur, can these professionals survive while maintaining a commitment to justice?

The Virtue of Justice

The virtue of justice is the strict habit of rendering what is due to others. Embodied in this brief definition, however, is one of the most complex of all the virtues. One reason for its complexity is that, unlike all the other virtues, it has no mean. Since all persons are assumed to possess fundamental dignity, and since human affairs are less than perfect even in the best of circumstances, it is impossible to be "too just." On the other hand, defects in rendering what is due to individuals and societies are abundant throughout human history. Much of the difficulty arising in public discussions about commutative or distributive justice can be found in this reality of justice and its lack of a mean. It is not obvious to anyone, as it might be with regard to intemperance or pusillanimity, or some of the extremes that are regulated by other virtues, what the proper balance due to individuals and groups might be. As a result, long, tortuous, bitter political disputes result. How does one compensate those whose ancestors were slaves? How does one right the inequities in a system that is constantly evolving? How much should be paid in awards to a person who now suffers as a consequence of a doctor's ineptitude?

These discussions, including the important issues of access to and rationing of health care, are always public ones, since they involve the common good. For this reason it is easy to forget that, at root, justice is a virtue about giving another individual, albeit a member of society, her due. There are three major elements of the virtue of justice: distributive, commutative, and rectificatory. Aristotle had expanded on earlier notions of the Greek philosophers that justice is the habit of giving another her due. He saw that a difference lay between giving one's due on grounds of the common good (distributive justice) and on grounds of individual good (rectificatory and commutative).[1] This insight enabled Aristotle to expand on another social virtue, friendship, arguing that it is right and good to love another person for his intrinsic goodness.[2] Later, St. Thomas Aquinas developed the virtue of justice further, and took from it insights about the social virtues and friendship that applied to the theological virtue of charity.[3] From this perspective, the social virtues acquired an additional impetus toward altruism not present in classical Greek thought. Somehow the ends of a good society dovetailed into a loving community in which God's presence would be found.

The determination to resolve international inequities, right the wrongs done to the environment, care for future generations, and foster peace are all part of the virtue of justice, whose voice, in Aquinas' view, is the altruism of agapeistic ethics.[4] Human rightness can never be sufficient. It is a far cry from the ideal community at any time in human history. St. Thomas, in his commentary on Job, puts the matter beautifully:

> Since their legislators cannot extend them to all singular cases, human laws are concerned with universal matters and with what occurs in most cases. How general human statutes are to be applied to individual deeds must be left to the prudence of the agent. As a result, man is open to many instances in which he falls short of rectitude, even though he does not run counter to human positive law.[5]

In a pluralistic society it is necessary to establish standards, developed and polished through constant discussion, as well as political and legislative action interpreted by the courts. These standards should be seen, however, as minimum requirements to give another her due. The reason for this is the already mentioned limitations on human wisdom; then, too, there are limits to benevolence, and there are conflicting claims and interpretations of the good. Precisely because we are conscious individuals acting with others in society, we must be committed, as Rawls claims, to act justly in concert about the common good.[6]

This is important, especially for the debate about access and rationing. Sometimes we are appalled by arguments that attempt to elevate to the maximum a minimalist understanding of human society and the social virtues. This minimalist move to the maximum tends to occur when one forgets that the root of justice lies in the individual's good, not only in the common good, in commutative as well as distributive justice.

We cannot do justice to the topic of justice in one chapter. Among the many issues with regard to the virtues are impartiality, the balance between treating equal persons equally and unequal persons unequally, relevant versus irrelevant issues, and the like. But we will explore the two major branches of the virtue here.

Commutative Justice

Our philosophy of medicine conflates commutative justice in the one-on-one situation with both the principle of beneficence and the virtue of benevolence, since we argue that in the doctor–patient relationship, the patient is due respect as a person such that the professional must always act on the basis of that person's good.

This is a secular, agapeistic, altruistic ethics grounded in the healing task. It cannot make sense in medicine to cure if one does not aim to heal the patient. Healing the patient requires exquisite attention to the medical good and to the patient's value system in which the good to be done is negotiated. We have called this "beneficence in trust," since it holds in trust the values of the patient during the negotiation about the actions to be done.[7]

The effort to do justice to the individual is both intelligent and a struggle. It requires intelligence to adjust continually to situations and to keep the other's needs and goods in view. As James Drane says:

> It is one thing to cultivate the urge for fairness; another to know what fairness is.
> All virtue involves the use of prudence and intelligence because virtues are refine-
> ments of human persons who cannot help but be in the world in an intelligent way.
> There is no such thing as blind virtue or ignorant virtue or unconscious virtue.[8]

Beyond intelligence, the virtue of justice involves a struggle. It is often a painful task to constantly adjust and balance conflicting needs and goods, especially if they are under our voluntary care. The task of equalizing or of being fair requires constant vigilance and monitoring. Calabresi and Bobbitt argue that despite any efforts made, human society inevitably creates tragic choices because the resources are always scarce and, in their words, "no general discussion can anticipate the various as-sociations, connotative and emotive, which the members of a society may attach to a particular good; hearts are different from livers."[9]

Duties Based on the Virtue of Justice

Current theories of justice, like the principle of beneficence itself, are transformed by a theory of the virtues. The notion of justice in contemporary theories is ultimately practical and prudential. We owe others their due because we want them to give us our due and because we want to protect ourselves from the unjust claims of others. Justice is a requirement for a peaceable society and the protection of legit-imate self-interest. If we practice justice, we can thereby ensure happiness for all. Justice, in this view, is a claim we have on the community—compliance with which is an obligation of communal living. In its highest expressions, it might be justified as owed to humans because they are worthy of respect and dignity.

On the view of the virtues, however, justice has its deepest roots in love; it is an extension of the charity we should show to others.[10] Not to do justice would be to relapse into self-interest, to turn from love of the other to love of self. Love testifies that the claims of others upon us are the claims of our brothers and sisters in a community of compassion and care. By that fact, individuals are entitled to be loved, especially in health care settings.

Love generates and transmutes justice. As St. Augustine held, justice is the concern and love that individuals in a community must show to others. Charity is for him "the root of all good."[11] It truly is the *vis a tergo* moving us to justice.

Justice energized by love transcends the legalistic justice of a chess-game approach to our duties to one another. Justice, therefore, expresses special concern for those in pain, the poor, the troubled, the oppressed, and the outcast. Justice transformed by communal concern is expressed in concrete acts of beneficence toward specific persons. Justice therefore is not only conformity with abstract principles. Such justice does not focus on strict interpretations of what is owed in accordance with some calculus of claims and counterclaims. Instead, it offers the way of love illuminated by a medical commitment to others. Medically driven justice does not rest solely on the virtue of justice itself, but modulates and illuminates it by a principle of a very different sort—the principle of beneficence in trust—and sometimes by a religious commitment to care for vulnerable individuals in a religious health care setting.[12] It is not only knowledge that generates justice, as in Plato or Aristotle, but the loving concern of the community of care itself.

The ways in which the classical construals of justice in Plato, Aristotle, and the Roman Stoics intersect with the notion we have just adumbrated are worthy of continuing examination. The same is true of the intersections with contemporary ethics. Frankena, for example, suggests that the ethics of love is a theory of its own—"pure agapeism."[13] Justice philosophically derived, and justice in a religious sense, cannot be fully equated. Their relationships and differences merit closer study in any attempt to determine whether or not, and how, purely religious notions of love and justice modify the ethics of health care. Just how the natural and supernatural virtues complement, supplement, or transform each other is a subject of its own, too.[14] It could be similarly argued on philosophical grounds that justice is ultimately rooted in benevolence and beneficence. In this way, love can be the first principle of naturalistic as well as of religious ethics. Only the former concerns us here, as philosophers.

It is the awareness of a call to all persons to live a life of love and compassion, and the conscious answer to this call, that for a physician transforms a profession into a vocation. This does not mean that higher orders of love and justice are not discernible to other professionals, or that physicians automatically practice these virtues. Rather, the medical profession means fidelity to a notion of justice transmuted by love and compassion as a moral obligation. Health care is one way of committing ourselves to the good of others, one way to respond to this call. With respect to this struggle of commutative justice and distributive justice, the most important problem in being fair is presented as a conflict about autonomy.

Conflicts of Autonomy and Justice

If the antimony between respect for autonomy and beneficence is more apparent than real, as we suggested in Chapter 4, this is not the case with autonomy and justice. Respecting the autonomy of the patient may inflict harm on third parties close to or distant from the patient. Here we face a fundamental dilemma of the idea of *prima facie* principles. When two such principles are in conflict, we must choose between them. To do so, one principle must eclipse the other. But how do we decide which one?

Justice is the most complex of the four principles and the only one that is simultaneously a virtue and a principle. As a virtue, it is a character trait, a habitual disposition to render to each person what is due. As a principle, it ordains that we act in such fashion that we render to each what is due her and that we treat like cases alike. There is, thus, an element of justice in each of the other principles, since we owe it to humans not to harm them, to respect their autonomy, and to do good when we can. Justice, therefore, has a certain prior status in determining the right and the good. In this sense, it limits the exercise of our own autonomy and our obligation to respect the autonomy of others. Justice, thus, sets limits on the absolutization of autonomy toward which the autonomy-based models of the doctor–patient relationship tend.

Some examples of cases in which respect for the autonomy of one person may impose injustice on another are these: the HIV-positive patient who refuses to disclose the fact to her sexual partners or persists in having unprotected sexual intercourse; the airline pilot or railroad engineer who refuses to disclose his substance abuse to his employer; the patient who demands marginally beneficial treatments that use up inordinate amounts of health care resources; and the psychiatric patient who intends to harm others.[15]

Respecting the patient's autonomy can also compromise the autonomy of the physician—not his autonomy to treat as he sees fit without reference to the patient's best interests, but his autonomy as a human being with personal values and beliefs. An example of this type are the demands of some patients, on grounds of patient autonomy, that the physician violate standards of good care to provide treatments that are scientifically dubious. Of like kind are demands that the physician perform abortion, participate in euthanasia, or withdraw artificial feeding and hydration when these actions would violate the physician's conscience.

Instances of this kind are increasing as the pressure to absolutize the individual's autonomy becomes more insistent. There is a growing sentiment in certain public and private quarters that the physician is merely the instrument of the patient's will. Some have even argued that the physician should leave personal morality behind in her professional life. In this view, not to provide what the patient wants, or what institutional policy or financial considerations dictate, is to violate not only the rule of autonomy but also beneficence and, indeed, justice. In this view, the physician's monopoly of medical knowledge is taken as a warrant to justify the patient's claim irrespective of the physician's values.

Judgments about how best to resolve the conflict between *prima facie* principles or, perhaps more accurately, individual interpretations of how those principles ought to be applied, are difficult. Justice has a trumping function in these conflicts. Under what circumstances should it take moral precedence over autonomy? These circumstances would obtain when there is a serious identifiable harm to a third party or parties and all other measures to protect autonomy have been taken. These conditions would be met in the case of the patient with HIV infection or the operators of public conveyances, where even a small possibility of grievous harm to others outweighs the claim to autonomy and preservation of confidentiality. The harm to others is more remote and less clearly identifiable in cases where patients demand dubious, marginal, or excessively costly treatments. Here the physician might more readily balance the psychological benefits to the patient against possible indefinite harm to others.

When the patient or social policy dictates that the physician submerge her own moral values to accommodate the patient's demands, even if what is demanded is accepted practice, then the conflict is between the patient's and the physician's autonomy. Here we must argue that the physician, no less than the patient, is a moral agent, that her autonomy is as deserving of respect as the patient's, and that justice would require that neither physician nor patient impose her values on the other. If it is maleficent to violate the autonomy of the patient, it is equally maleficent to violate that of the physician.

In practical terms, this will mean that, institutionally and ethically, mechanisms must be devised to permit physicians as well as patients to withdraw from their relationship. This must be done amicably, respectfully, and only after another physician has agreed to accept the transfer of responsibility for the care of the patient. The physician cannot withdraw without first making provisions for transfer to another physician because to do so would constitute abandonment, in itself a serious breach of ethical obligation rooted in the virtue of justice and the principle of beneficence.

Social Justice: The Challenge of Decent Health Care

One of the most difficult problems of distributive justice is that of providing decent and fair health care for all citizens. Current distributive challenges to a decent health care system will now be considered.

Resources

There is a lack of adequate resources to care for many people. Today there are 38 million underinsured and uninsured persons in the United States, and this number is projected to increase to 50 million underinsured in the 1990s. Some states reimburse for Medicaid and Medicare expenses so slowly that hospitals quickly run out of money and are forced to close.[16]

The State of Illinois at the end of April 1988 ran out of funding for Medicaid. All poor persons to be treated by hospitals from that date until the end of the fiscal year had to be treated at the largesse of institutions and health care providers.

Entrepreneurship

Entrepreneurship drives health professionals to make excessive profits from the illness of others. Such marketing of health care drives professionals toward paying patients and highly profitable ventures and away from caring for the chronically ill, the dispossessed and homeless, AIDS patients, and the like. Criticism has been leveled against a former NIH researcher-physician who took the discovering of interleuken-2, based on years of taxpayer-funded research, and formed a company for treating end-stage cancer patients with this new therapy.[17] Recently, Lutheran General Hospital in Park Ridge, Illinois, contracted with this company to provide the special cancer care, even though another major medical center in the Chicago area already provides it.

Engelhardt and Rie argue that a modern secular state should not and cannot regulate for-profit corporations in health care and that all medical care, except for explicitly offered charity care, has some element of the commodity. They claim that it would be hard to conceive a moral basis for regulating the sale of health care. Part of this claim rests on the changing character of modern health care, in which physicians are no longer responsible entirely to their patients, but rather must include social and public responsibility to third-party payers. They conclude, as we did in another work, that patients must be told if conflicts of responsibility are possible.[18,19] But another part of the claim rests on the notion that it may be a "virtue" that for-profit corporations skim and dump. Skimming is the practice of taking only the best patients (those who can pay) and not treating the poor. Dumping is the practice of transferring indigent patients from private to public institutions purely for economic reasons. The authors argue that these all too common practices are good, both because they force society to own up to its responsibilities to the poor and because they underline the (by implication) nasty practice of asking those who can pay for their health care to subsidize those who cannot. As they say:

> It [skimming] forces the public to recognize that in the absence of skimming, those who can pay are subject to an informal tax, a shifting of costs, to provide care to those who cannot pay. . . . Skimming compels individuals, communities, and governments to confront the question of the level of care they wish to provide the indigent.[20]

We agree that public policy about levels of care is an important and urgent issue. But the authors assume that it is somehow immoral to ask the community, without its explicit and voting consent, to care for others. This is a direct consequence of Engelhardt's (and, we presume, Rie's) libertarian view of the community, a view that is fatally flawed from the point of view of almost any perspective.[21] Nothing more clearly shows the fundamental clash of values between an autonomy-based theory and a community-based theory than to call skimming and dumping the "virtues of skimming and dumping."[22]

Gatekeeping

Gatekeeping places health professionals in a new, alien, and ambivalent relation with patients. Gatekeeping forces health professionals to become wall-eyed. One eye is on the good the patient, and the other is on the good of the institution, HMO, or society itself. This raises questions about the primacy of social obligations *versus* caring for individual patients.

Although a national consensus is building for reform of the health care system, it still remains a very complex political, public policy, and ethical issue. With good reason. Virtually alone among advanced countries, the United States does not yet consider it a right for all citizens to have equal access to health care. Other problems with the system make it creak and groan in comparison with the delivery systems of other countries. At the very least, basic health care coverage for all is a desirable goal of any decent human society. It is not just unfortunate that millions of us have no access to health care and that the middle class often can no longer afford it. Rather it is unjust, since not providing it has been an act of political will.

There are many causes of the continued upward spiral of costs that contribute to the sense of crisis about our health care system. For as the costs continue to rise at twice the inflation rate, every one of us suffers from decreased access, loss of jobs in society due to lack of competitively priced products, increased copayment in insurance plans, and the like. Industry in the United States is spending almost half of its profits on health care, compared with 7% in 1960.[23] Unions are cast in the role of protesting cuts in benefits because they thought they had contracted for lifetime health care benefits.[24]

Some of these cost-contributing causes are impervious to straightforward political resolution. Rather, the causes are driven by the inherent value system of medicine and health care technology. Good examples are the proliferation of institutionalization of health care since the 1950s and the expansion of concomitant subspecialties.[25] Another cause is the intrinsic law of technological development, which suggests constant improvement and progress rather than stability as a fundamental value. As a result, pictures in promotional literature, magazines, and newspapers tend to show happy specialists and administrators outside the newest 7-ton magnet for the MRI rather than happy home-care nurses helping elderly citizens live partially independent lives in their own environments. The latter is too stable and time-tested to catch our eye. The former is sexy and exciting. And costly!

Nonetheless, reform is coming, since economic self-interest will always win the day. Before we begin any flag-waving about reforms, however, we should recognize that the desire to reform stems from two major competing interests. Some support for reform arises from high-minded principles of justice, while other support stems from a desire to control costs. Many countries have been able to combine both interests in reasonable plans, but it is difficult. How may we provide greater coverage at less cost? If we do not succeed, our products will become even less competitive on the world market and access to health care for all citizen will diminish at an even greater pace than it does today.

Even granting one or the other of the two competing interests, there is widespread disagreement among parties within each of these opposing camps. Consider the different notions of justice that drive alternate proposals for rationing and/or access by many of our colleagues. Or think of the schemes for controlling costs that clash with one another: cut benefits, cut bureaucracy, eliminate government from the doctor–patient relationship, establish more governmental control of costs, provide "chits" for private purchase of insurance, and so on.

Two obvious reasons for lowering costs are to eliminate waste, paperwork, and intermediaries from the health care environment and to control runaway malpractice costs. Little hope remains that the American propensity to sue will be kept in check or that the right to sue, like the right to keep and bear arms, will at any time be abridged. Ironically, the constant pressure on the health care system this propensity creates becomes entirely self- and community-destructive. The first impetus will most likely take the form of government contracts with one or several insurance companies to provide all-inclusive care for all citizens. Colorado has proposed this method of providing access to care for all. In essence this is a modification of the

Canadian scheme, which is not, as critics would have it, a socialized medicine plan. Rather, a single insurance agency provides the care, and that agency is controlled by government so that costs can be controlled.

The Special Case of the Elderly

As gerification of society continues, disruptions are caused in the community. Some, like Daniel Callahan, argue that society must cut off its high-technology medicine past a certain age.[26] Yet setting limits on the basis of age, or the opportunity to compete for goods and resources, or any other external criterion introduces philosophical and procedural difficulties, not the least of which is the commitment to give persons their due that anchors social justice in individual good.

For one thing, we must establish what will count as basic care and what portion of that care will be mandated in the health care system.[27] Prominent thinkers, too, have proposed limiting care on the basis of age. Yet this position seems morally indefensible and, according to Baruch Brody, unworkable.[28] It is unworkable because of the problem of "identifiable lives." It is one thing to work out on paper a system of allocation on the basis of age; it is quite another to accept that rationing scheme when a family member is involved.[29] General, more abstract principles might make sense logically. But when an identified individual suffers, the abstract principles become unpopular and unacceptable.[30]

In addition to problems with proposals like the ones by Lamm, Callahan,[31] Veatch, and Engelhardt (less so with Daniels),[32,33] there are problems with the orientation of the health care system itself, which Jesse Jackson terms the "sick-care system." This orientation "sets" limits as well, although they are invisible standards built into the delivery mechanisms and DRGs.[34] Each proposal represents not inconsiderable minds tackling not inconsiderable problems.[35,36] Yet many of them share one feature: an objective, permanent limit on access.

A system of access ought to be designed that permits the following features to emerge:

- Floating limits, so that the doctor–patient relationship and its flexibility remain intact. Individual needs and treatment plans would then continue to be made possible.
- Equal treatment of all persons in the same categories of illness, regardless of social status, ability to pay for additional care, and so on. This is our objection to the Oregon Plan, since it focuses only on the poor, while others who can pay would get access to limited-benefit care.[37]
- Physician involvement in defining the limits of care to be provided, through research and practice experience with medically indicated treatments for specific conditions.
- Some public control, nonetheless, on spiraling health care costs.
- Emphasis on advance decisions by all persons regarding their care.
- Annual review of medical advances and provision for effective treatments included in the flexible plan noted.

- Emphasis on wellness and prevention, and on quality of life over prolonging life. This can be accomplished by changing certain default modes of treatment now in place.
- Awareness that care for the elderly is part of a social revolution that will be required in the just community, free of age discrimination.

Floating Limits

To set limits, as Larry Churchill suggests, is inimical to the American spirit. Our vision of rugged individualism and limitless frontiers to conquer, our crusades of mercy, our wars on poverty, our social commitments despite a halting form of social justice are all examples of that spirit. Nowhere is the idea of establishing boundaries on care more repugnant than when considering care for the elderly.[38] The social vision of caring for the elderly is an important part of the kind of society we want to be. Every person wants to be needed. No one should feel like unnecessary baggage that slows down the social machine. This deeper vision of social concern about the elderly can be detected in our original legislative goals for caring for the elderly.

But these legislative goals, and the vision that animated them, have largely vanished. In their place is increasing social pressure to limit access to health care on the basis of age. The social contract itself may have to change precisely because of an aging citizenry.[39] The temptation to allocate all social goods, not just health care, on the basis of age is enormous.

The problem with each proposal for limits is that it cannot be based on a "natural" criterion. As Erich Loewy has argued, the "natural lifespan" of Callahan is not only wrong but also impossible to describe. It will change as our abilities in health care change. One of the reasons age cutoffs appear so abhorrent is that an elderly person in Callahan's category of 80 years of age (say, a man like Bob Hope, who still golfs) might need arthroscopic surgery to remove painful bone chips in his shoulder. Why should he be denied this surgery? Our instincts tell us that his "natural" life span is considerably extended and may be more so in the future if genetic manipulation and prevention mechanisms continue to develop rapidly. Indeed, in the next century, it may be possible to give birth to a generation of human beings who will have to choose to die.

The reason argumentation alone cannot confront the problem of ageist proposals is that nothing short of a social revolution will be able to address the massive numbers of elderly people who will need some support in the future. Recall the demographics. Within fifty years, the number of dependent people will increase almost tenfold. A leading authority writes: "There is no hope of carrying the burden of old age that the future has in store without assistance from the family and neighbors at least equal to that given at the present time."[40] This burden will require a rethinking of the goals of human life (e.g., not retirement in Florida, but taking care of elderly parents in a mother-in-law wing of one's house in Chicago). It also challenges us to reshape our conception of the community as a community of healers. Thus, what is needed is a social revolution because it requires rethinking of the freedoms we normally assign to one another.

As we have already noted in discussing the conflict between justice and autonomy, the role of self-determination in a major social policy designed to care for all citizens is important. The primary point is to underscore ways in which individuals might gain more control over expensive medical technology. While aiding themselves and their values, they also assist society in controlling costs and diminish, but not eliminate, the impact of rationing.

Little can be gained by assuming simplistic postures about any one of the incredibly complex issues that do arise when technology meets human life. But there does seem to be a difference between issues at the beginning of life and those at the end of life, of obstetrical and pediatric issues compared to geriatric ones. In the former instances, we are dealing with potential persons. Although such beings have human rights, they may be more restricted legally than those of fully functioning human beings. Thus, a frozen embryo might, in the future, acquire the right to be implanted (as it apparently now has in Australia), but not, of course, the rights of free speech, assembly, suffrage, and the like, that we honor in moral persons (those who are able to make moral choices).

At the end of life, by contrast, we are considering persons who have constructed a value history. Even if a few pediatric and geriatric patients are now considered incompetent, there is a world of difference between them.

The heart of the difference lies in the fulfillment of the capacity to make decisions, either upon values we already have or upon values that emerge after reflection on the decision. Although all beings should be valued by us and their integrity preserved as far as possible, when a tragic choice is forced on us, it is far easier to make a decision about applying a medical technology or withholding it altogether based on values constructed by a patient over a lifetime than on a "valueless" field presented by the embryo or newborn. At least in theory, debates about the living will and other forms of controlling the application of medical technologies to the end of life should be less intense than those about abortion and the care of defective newborns. Honoring the values of the individual as part of decisions to be made about them once they are incompetent is the primary way we can respect their inherent dignity. If they are dying, we should never strip them of the lifetime of choices their values represent.

A position of solid commitment to the value of human life, even that which may no longer be a moral person as we normally understand personhood, produces the safest insurance against bigotry, repression, neo-Nazism, and murder. This position becomes a truism if there is no attempt to define the kinds of efforts that will be required in directing technology. Some important examples are worth discussing.

Life Prolongation

As the staggering statistics about an increasingly elderly population become a reality and our children become a problem for our grandchildren, extremely sophisticated norms for withholding and withdrawing expensive forms of care will have to be established. These will probably be based on current guidelines that cover terminal illness, but the major ethical and legal issues today surround disputes about certain conditions, such as advanced Alzheimer's disease or a permanent coma, that may or may not be seen as terminal states. The congressional study by the Office of Technology Assessment is helpful in this regard, as it enumerates the areas in which the application of technology to the elderly causes both ethical and economic problems.[41]

Controlling life-prolonging technologies is but one aspect of the larger problem of directing technology to human aims. Nowhere is this more apparent than in the application of medical technology and its various interventions to the aging and dying patient. There is a fallacy in thinking that everyone wants the very "best" medical technology. The fallacy involved equates technology with better care. Not surprisingly, studies have confirmed that it is not the technology but the care persons receive that determines their well-being, and in the case of elderly patients, the protection of their human spirit to the end. Dramatic changes in health care also have changed what was once more personal and familial care. There has been an enormous increase in the technologization of care. Where once a cold compress might have been applied and one's hands held, now all sorts of interventions are possible, from intravenous fluids and nutrition, blood products and agents to prevent clotting or bleeding, and cardiopulmonary resuscitation to experimental treatments such as advanced chemotherapeutic agents, radiologic implants, artificial hearts, and transplants of other organs. For the most part, these interventions are much better than a cold compress. But to the extent that personal control over the process of dying is lost, new protections must be developed. Following *Cruzan,* a living will strengthens the advance directive a patient gives about his or her care. As we will examine the problems associated with advance directives in Chapter 15, we will not discuss them further here, except to note that a virtuous individual is required to interpret these directives in light of the good of the patient and the healing aims of medicine.

The Social Good

The justice issues are largely confined to academic discussion until voters make their concerns known. Presidential candidates tout their own versions of such reform, as do senators and congressmen and women. In the midst of the politics, it is easy to forget that health care is a good and a service prerequisite for the well-being of all human beings. In earlier times, the essential moral quality of health care was embedded in the professional codes of the caregivers themselves, largely physicians and nurses. With the rise of modern technological health care, the former one-on-one relationship between doctor and patient became institutionalized. Hospitals were no longer like hotels where physicians signed their patients in-and-out at will. Suddenly, with escalating costs and the subsequent social and political monitoring, the doctor–patient relation became a provider–patient one, with government, third-party payers, institutions themselves, and myriad other specialists and ancillary caregivers counted as well. All of these players have complementary and sometimes competing interests in the reform of the health system as well.

This radical transformation of the original doctor–patient relationship has created a sense of chaos and loss of control, especially over essential values in caring for individuals in our society. There are some overriding ethical considerations in the design of any national health program. The first must be that the patients ought to have control over their care, so that they do not experience difficulties and delays in obtaining appropriate and approved treatment. The second is that the moral character of the institutions of health delivery and of the practitioners of health care are not destroyed through bureaucratic requirements. The third ethical consideration is that, since some form of rationing will be required regarding specific treatments to be made available, the national health program itself should be designed to be as efficient as possible. This means that greater effort must be made than heretofore to fund patient care rather than administrative overhead costs. Fourth, the quality of human judgement and flexibility in treating individual differences should be maintained as far as possible, so that formulaic responses to human pain and misery are avoided. Otherwise, treating people with respect will diminish.

Modern health care is a unique melding of charity and business, of compassion and attention to fiscal responsibility. If health care institutions are required to maintain this delicate balance, so too should the national health program that emerges from political debate. Incentives to hold down costs and to increase the quality of care should be built into the plan. But so too should incentives to cooperate rather than compete, to ensure commitment to patients and their values, as well as the survival of institutions. No institution should benefit by shunning essential care. Sharing the burden of expensive and unreimbursed care among institutions also ought to be designed into the national health program. This will still be required, since not all health care interventions will be covered under any conceivable program.

How did the health care crisis come about? It is insufficient to cite failures in public health or preventive medicine. The very successes of modern medicine have also caused disruptions. Failures as well as successes have caused the loss of institutional identity. Consider the problem of the gerification of society. This problem is almost directly caused by the successes of control of infectious disease and the suppression of the effects of high blood pressure. Major interventions such as open-heart surgery, insulin treatment, and cancer chemotherapy are also aids in helping people live longer.

But as gerification continues, disruptions are caused in the community. Some, like Daniel Callahan, argue that society must cut off its high-technology medicine past a certain age.[42]

The Physician–Patient Relationship

In the changed sociopolitical, economic, and scientific climates in which medicine is practiced today, there are conflicting conceptions of **the healing relationship**. Elsewhere we have sketched a religious phenomenological analysis of the healing relationship.[43] Some of the formulations of this relationship would be more congenial to a philosophical perspective than others. Thus, it would not require a faith commitment to discern that a biological model of the physician–patient or healing relationship would be insufficient, if not antithetic to, a more complete interpretation of healing or helping. The same could be said of the relationship viewed as a legal contract, a commodity relationship, or a strongly paternalistic one. Other models—the covenantal, friendship, or fidelity to promise—would be more congruent with a compassionate sense of the virtue of justice.[44]

All the models cited have some verisimilitude. Without denying this fact, it is the model perceived as primary that is of the utmost importance, the one that takes precedence over the others. Thus, strong paternalism would rarely, if ever, be countenanced, while weak paternalism could be.[45] A strictly libertarian relationship would not be consistent, since it would forbid intervention in suicide or euthanasia, for example. With these exceptions, respect for the autonomy of the patient as a human being would not only be consistent but required. So, too, would respect for the respective agency of patient and physician, with neither imposing on the other except where grave harm was in prospect. There would also be a strong imperative to mutual respect for the personal moral accountability of both the physician and the patient. Neither could ask the other to act contrary to conscience, a feature sometimes lacking in contemporary accounts of justice.

Likewise, a strictly contractual model of **the healing relationship** is insufficient from a loving perspective on justice. The contractual model requires only a minimalistic ethic—one that obligates the patient and the physician to fulfill the terms of an agreement and nothing more. This model calls for the minimal amount of beneficence. It is contrived to reduce dependence upon either the physician's benevolence or his fidelity to promises. It is precisely those features of the relationship that a contract cannot cover—the uncertainties inherent in the clinical situation and reliance on the fidelity and good will of the physician and patient that a loving justice most clearly regulates.

The most distinctive characteristic of **a healing relationship** motivated by loving justice is the higher degree of self-effacement it requires as a matter of course. Even on strictly philosophical grounds, the vulnerability of the sick person imposes a special responsibility not to take advantage of the patient. In a more positive sense, the physician becomes committed to some suppression of self-interest, comfort, and preferences in order to serve the patient. This is that "higher degree of self-effacement" that Harvey Cushing called the "common devotion" that should motivate the medical profession.[46]

Conclusion

Health care institutions can be said to have a conscience. This is a convenient shorthand for the sum total of their mission and commitments. Individuals within institutions, including the doctors practicing there, should both have a say in the formation of the mission and values statement of the institution and commit themselves to the mission and values. If administrators try to arrange for the care of individuals without health care insurance, then doctors with admitting privileges might be asked to help. If they refuse, should they be allowed to continue to have such privileges if their refusal violates a commitment of the institution and its leaders and staff?

Executives and staff ought to discuss and formulate policy positions so that they can contribute to the national debate about the outline, design, and implementation of a national health program. Some questions might be: If basic care is to be provided, what would not be covered? What sort of rationing plan would be most just? Should there be rationing? If so, can the public be urged to discuss different proposals for rationing that might be considered just? Should not one's own institution be part of that public discussion? What leadership might it provide?

These are not just strategic questions. They represent the moral center in justice of the enterprise that is health care delivery.

Notes

1. Aristotle, *Nicomachean Ethics,* V, 1–7, 1129a1–1135a14.

2. Ibid., VIII–IX, 1155a1–1172a15.

3. Thomas Aquinas, *Summa Theologiae,* 2, 2a, qq. 57–80.

4. G. B. Phelan, "Justice and Friendship," *The Thomist: The Maritain Volume, Dedicated to Jacques Maritain on the Occasion of His Sixtieth Anniversary* (New York: Sheed & Ward, 1943), pp. 153–170.

5. St. Thomas Aquinas, *Expositio in Job,* c. 11, lect. 1; *Parmenides,* XIV, 49; see Vernon Bourke, "Foundations of Justice," *Proceedings of the American Catholic Philosophical Association* 36 (1962):19–28.

6. John Rawls, *A Theory of Justice* (Cambridge, MA: Belknap Press of Harvard University Press, 1971).

7. Edmund D. Pellegrino and David C. Thomasma, *For the Patient's Good: The Restoration of Beneficence in Health Care* (New York: Oxford University Press, 1988).

8. James Drane, *Becoming a Good Doctor: The Place of Virtue and Character in Medical Ethics* (Kansas City, MO: Sheed & Ward and the Catholic Health Association, 1988), p. 106.

9. Guido Calabresi and Philip Bobbitt, *Tragic Choices: The Conflicts Society Confronts in the Allocation of Tragically Scarce Resources* (New York: Norton, 1978), p. 150.

10. Edmund D. Pellegrino and David C. Thomasma, *The Christian Virtues in Medicine,* Unpublished manuscript.

11. St. Augustine, *Fathers of the Church* (Sermon 73.4) as cited in William J. Walsh and John P. Langan, "Patristic Social Consciousness—the Church and the Poor," *The Faith that Does Justice,* ed. John C. Haughey. (New York: Paulist Press, 1977).

12. The question about the continuity or discontinuity of the supernatural and the natural virtues is still an intriguing one. Robert Sokowloski has examined this relationship in a brilliant monograph, illuminating both kinds of virtue. See his *The God of Faith and Reason* (Notre Dame, IN.: University of Notre Dame Press, 1982).

13. William Frankena, *Ethics,* 2d ed. (Englewood Cliffs, NJ: Prentice-Hall, 1973).

14. Pellegrino and Thomasma, *Christian Virtues.*

15. J. C. Beck (ed.), *Confidentiality versus the Duty to Protect: Foreseeable Harm in the Practice of Psychiatry* (Washington, DC: American Psychiatric Press, 1990).

16. One hospital in Chicago, Providence, closed its doors after owing over $48 million to creditors. The major reason for this debt was slow reimbursement by the state for care for the poor.

17. See Glenn C. Graber, and David C. Thomasma, *Theory and Practice in Medical Ethics* (New York: Continuum, 1989): pp. 186–188.

18. H. Tristram Engelhardt, Jr., and Michael A. Rie, "Morality for the Medical-Industrial Complex: A Code of Ethics for the Mass Marketing of Health Care," *New England Journal of Medicine* 319(16) (October 20, 1988):1086–1089.

19. Pellegrino and Thomasma, *For the Patient's Good*.

20. Engelhardt and Rie, "Medical-Industrial Complex," p. 1088.

21. In fact, Erich H. Loewy shows how Engelhardt's view of the ethical foundations is flawed from a secular point of view of the community as well in his review of *The Foundations of Bioethics,* "Not By Reason Alone: A Review of Engelhardt's *Foundations of Bioethics,*" *Journal of Medical Humanities and Bioethics* 8(1) (January, 1987):67–72. Also see E. H. Loewy, "The Role of Suffering and Community in Clinical Ethics," *Journal of Clinical Ethics* 2(2) (Summer, 1991):83–89.

22. Engelhardt and Rie, "Medical-Industrial Complex," p. 1087.

23. See "Industry Spends Almost Half of Profits on Health Care: A Report on 'Future of Corporate Health Benefits: A National Report'," *Loyola World* (August 27, 1992):9.

24. "Unions Protest Navistar Bid to Cut Health Benefits," *Chicago Tribune* (August 12, 1992):Section 3, p. 3.

25. Carlos J. M. Martini, "Graduate Medical Education in the Changing Environment of Medicine," *Journal of the American Medical Association* 268(9) (September 2, 1992):1097–1105.

26. Daniel Callahan, *Setting Limits: Medical Goals in an Aging Society* (New York: Simon & Schuster, 1987).

27. Fredrick R. Abrams, "The Basis of Basic Care," *Frontlines* 7(2) (October 1990): 2, 11.

28. Baruch A. Brody, "The Macro-Allocation System of Health Care Resources," *Health Care Systems: Moral Conflicts in European and American Public Policy,* ed. Hans-Martin Sass and Robert U. Massey (Dordrecht: Kluwer, 1988), pp. 213–236.

29. E. Haavi Morreim, "Fiscal Scarcity and the Inevitability of Bedside Budget Balancing," *Archives of Internal Medicine* 149(5) (May 1989):1012–1015.

30. Norman Daniels, "Why Saying 'No' to Patients in the United States Is So Hard," *The New England Journal of Medicine* 314 (May 22, 1986):1380–1383.

31. Callahan, *Setting Limits*.

32. Norman Daniels, "Is Age Rationing Just?", *Efficacy in Health Care: Essays from the First International Conference on Justice in Health Care,* ed. Andrew Griffin (Chicago: Illinois Masonic Hospital, 1990), pp. 11–22.

33. Norman Daniels, *Am I My Parents' Keeper? An Essay on Justice Between the Young and the Old* (New York: Oxford University Press, 1988).

34. Leonard M. Fleck, "DRGs: Justice and the Invisible Rationing of Health Care Resources," *Journal of Medicine and Philosophy* 12(2) (May 1987):165–196.

35. Leonard M. Fleck, "Just Health Care (I): Is Beneficence Enough?" *Theoretical Medicine* 10(2) (June 1989):167–182.

36. Ibid., 299–308.

37. Lisa Holton, "The Oregon Answer: A Radical Experiment in the Name of Rationing," *American College of Physicians Observer* 10(6) (June 1990):11.

38. Larry Churchill, *Rationing Health Care in America: Perceptions and Principles of Justice* (Notre Dame, IN: University of Notre Dame Press, 1987), p. 20.

39. C. M. Madigan, "As Citizenry Ages, Social Contract May Have to Change," *Chicago Tribune* (August 27, 1989):Section 4, p. 1.

40. J. H. Sheldon, *British Journal of Medicine* (1950):1, 319.

41. Congress of the United States: *Office of Technology Assessment Brief 1987* (Washington, DC: U.S. Government Printing Office, 1987).

42. Daniel Callahan, *Setting Limits*.

43. Edmund D. Pellegrino and David C. Thomasma, *Health and Healing* (in press in Italian translation).

44. See William F. May, *The Physician's Covenant* (Philadelphia: Westminster Press, 1983); Pedro Lain Entralgo, *La relacion medico-enfermo, historia y teoria* (Madrid: Revista De Occidente, 1964), pp. 235–258; and E. D. Pellegrino, "Toward a Reconstruction of Medical Morality: The Primacy of the Act of Profession and the Fact of Illness," *Journal of Medicine and Philosophy* 4(1)(March 1979):32–56.

45. See James Childress' discussion of strong and weak paternalism in his *Who Should Decide? Paternalism in Health Care* (New York: Oxford University Press, 1982), pp. 102–112.

46. Harvey Cushing, "The Common Devotion," *Consecratio Medici and Other Papers* (Boston: Little, Brown, 1929), pp. 3–13.

9

Fortitude

The virtue of fortitude is often considered to be coextensive with courage. The words can be interchanged depending on the context. But in this chapter, we will use the term "courage" to describe the more physical aspects of the virtue, for example, the courage of a fireman entering a burning building, or of Evil Knievel hurtling out over a canyon in his motorcycle. Fortitude, on the other hand, will represent moral courage, for example, the willingness of an individual to suffer personal harm for the sake of a moral good, the spy who does not reveal potentially destructive secrets to an enemy, or the hostage who faces the daily terror of loneliness and isolation.

Our interest in this chapter is in how a society that focuses so much on physical courage—indeed, it is the warp and woof of most of our television programs and movie dramas—tends to neglect moral courage or fortitude. This neglect is especially problematic for the physician.

General Consideration of Fortitude

A look at the classical exploration of fortitude reveals the possibility of making a distinction between moral and physical courage. Fortitude is not considered to be coextensive with courage. Rather, one might consider fortitude to be sustained courage. It has a note of constancy to it that singular courageous acts may not have. *Webster's Dictionary* defines fortitude as "firm courage; patient endurance of misfortune, pain, etc."[1] As in all the virtues, the emphasis is on sustainability—not on individual and isolated acts, but on the disposition to act continuously in a certain way.

Courage, as Plato saw, may exist in otherwise evil persons.[2] He often notes that too much courage is apt to make persons bestial, and that it must be tempered with moderation.[3] Other notes are ones of "remaining at one's post in face of adversity"[4] and of bravery, constancy, and valor. In general, there is a military cast to the virtue as described by Plato. Persons having too much courage might have been military persons who killed without mercy and "went berserk." That is not what we mean by fortitude. Courage, instead, should not be seen as synonymous with macho behavior. Courage may consist of temperate responses when all around us are urging precipitate actions. The virtue also encompasses resistance to retreat from the right thing to do in the face of corporate, collegial, or public adversity.

Given the general theory of virtue held by Aristotle, the virtue of fortitude could not be found in an evil person. His account of the virtues holds that the virtues are a special character trait, a *"hexis* of character."[5] For Aristotle the virtues concern our responses to our feelings. Feelings themselves have no moral qualities; they just are. Rather, the moral quality is acquired from the person's trained response to feelings of anger, outrage, fear, dread, and so on. This trained response becomes a character trait when one can predict a disposition to act in a certain way toward those feelings.[6] Aristotle says of training: "what is trained is something which, by being changed repeatedly in a certain way by guidance which is not innate, is eventually capable of acting in that way."[7] For Aristotle the individual who is trained to be courageous would also choose to be virtuous in other spheres. The important point about "excellence of character" (*arete*) is that it is a matter of choice. One chooses to act on feelings and natural inclinations in a certain way, and one chooses to be disposed in this way as well. In short, the virtues control the natural impulses of personality and circumstances, toward goodness.

Hence when St. Thomas Aquinas, following Aristotle, asks whether there are many moral virtues or just one, he answers in part:

> . . . in moral matters man's reasonable part holds the place of commander and mover, while his emotional part is commanded and moved. Yet the appetite does not receive the action of reason as it were univocally, for it is rational not essentially but by participation, as we read in the *Ethics*. Accordingly as under the control of reason its objects are established in various species by having various relations to reason. The consequence is that virtues are of various species, and are not just one.[8]

Thus the unity of prudence, and of the moral life, depends on the singleness of the object. As we have pointed out, the object of all the moral virtues is to provide both an intensity of choice and a balance between extremes of appetite.

There are many examples of this virtuous control over one's personality in human history: the Buddha, Jesus, St. Augustine, St. Dominic, St. Teresa of Avila. Each of these individuals faced enormous challenges and inner struggles. It was said of St. Ignatius of Loyola that he never lost his serenity, either in adversity or in joy. This was a remarkable characteristic of his leadership. But this character trait was a result of years of struggle with his personality, years of choosing to maintain his imperturbability instead of giving his personality free expression.

The virtue of fortitude or courage concerns the feelings of fear and of confidence. In Aristotle's view, all the virtues are concerned with a disposition to choose the mean between two extremes; the extreme feelings to be avoided are cowardice, on the one hand, and rashness, on the other. Not stirring the waters is cowardice because it leaves patients without advocacy. But stirring the waters too much and too publicly is rashness, which is counterproductive. So Aristotle cautions that "courage is a mean with respect to things that inspire confidence or fear . . . and it chooses or endures things because it is noble to do so, or because it is base not to do so."[9] So it would be cowardly to escape from poverty or pain by committing suicide, not a virtue of fortitude. Fortitude endures such things.

For St. Thomas, fearlessness is actually a vice, since it eliminates the natural fear one should have in the face of a difficulty. He was fond of quoting Aristotle to the effect that virtue concerns what is both difficult and good.[10] What is difficult is the pressure of our feelings that might overwhelm us from time to time. Since courage essentially controls our fears that would lead us from flight, Aquinas wonders whether the virtuous person would totally eliminate these feelings:

> The Stoics debarred anger and all other feelings from the mind of the wise or virtuous man. But the Peripatetics, led by Aristotle, allowed the pressure of anger and other feelings in virtuous men provided that they were governed by reason.[11]

Aquinas, too, considered courage to be a cardinal virtue, like St. Gregory, St. Ambrose, and St. Augustine, who also commented on the importance of this virtue in one's moral life. The reason it is called such is that within it is found common characteristics of all the virtues. The common characteristic of courage for St. Thomas, as well as for Aristotle,[12] is *steadfast action:*

> It is courage which chiefly claims praise for steadfastness. He who firmly stands his ground is accorded greater praise in proportion to the pressure he withstands, which would force him to fall or retreat. Both pleasurable good and oppressive evil constrain a man to abandon reason. . . . [13]

The proper action of courage, then, is enduring and staunchness.[14]

As Drane argues, however, the virtues do not only order the inner moral life and contribute to one's character as a professional; they also assist individuals to discover the moral dimensions of reality. A good doctor is one who perceives the fears of the patient and tries to alleviate them, whereas a poor doctor may not recognize these fears at all. Drane continues:

> Virtues (or vices) structure character. They could be called orientations of character in the sense of balanced, rational patterns of choosing, feeling, and acting in accordance with ideals and standards of goodness communicated by a vision. Virtues are not the whole of ethics, but they contribute to good behavior, good persons, and even to good societies.[15]

A summary of these general considerations of courage and fortitude leads to the distinction between physical and moral courage. Physical courage is the virtue that renders a subject able to resist flight in the face of physical danger or moderates rash behavior under the same circumstances. A courageous general, for example, would neither retreat too early nor fail to retreat and lose all his men needlessly. Physicians today need a measure of physical courage if they minister to patients in warfare under fire, in a civil emergency, in going to an area of epidemics, or in treating persons with AIDS.

Moral courage, or fortitude, is the virtue that renders an individual capable of acting on principle in the face of potential harmful consequences without either retreating too soon from that principle or remaining steadfast to the point of absurdity. One can readily discern the requirements of balanced judgment and prudence in such situations. Physicians need fortitude to do the right thing when it is required and expected of them, given their role in life. In the ordinary practice of medicine, it is moral courage or fortitude in the face of consensus, rather than physical courage, that is depreciated by our society. We have too great an obsession with physical courage to the detriment of moral courage. If "everybody is doing it," how far should a physician resist on principle?

Let us look now at the way in which fortitude is a virtue that affects the public affairs of the physician.

Fortitude as a Medical Virtue

Perhaps no other virtue, with the possible exception of temperance, is harder to practice in today's environment than fortitude. The reason is that so much of the original freedom to practice medicine without constraints, a freedom that drew powerful individualists into the profession, has now been eroded not only by governmental and third-party rules, but also by community expectations.

By now, the litany of woes introduced by government and third-party regulation is familiar. In efforts to control costs, and sometimes but not often to increase access to inexpensive care, government has developed regulations and reimbursement formulae that have both positive and negative effects. Among the positive effects are at least modest gains in controlling costs by controlling what health care providers will receive for services. Among the negative effects, however, are loss of professional freedom; refusal to treat the poor and the elderly on Medicaid and Medicare, since reimbursement rarely measures up to the cost of providing it; and the emergence of ever more tightly managed structures for the practice of medicine. The latter concern us here.

The sheer weight of the bureaucracy that has sprung up around the regulations of health care providers has forced some physicians to sell their practices to hospitals or other health organizations. In these "vertically managed" systems, the physician appears once again free to practice medicine, required only to fill a certain quota of patients, while the corporation does the billing and collecting of funds and pays the physician.

Due to these and other widespread social changes, community expectations about the role of physicians have also changed. In times past, the community expected physicians to make individual judgments on the basis of the patient's best interests. Now the expectation is one of balance, often of conflicting values presented by patients, the community, and society itself.

To act courageously in such an environment of "corporate medicine" will become more and more difficult. There is increasing demand for physicians who are "team players," people who can function well in the environment of HMOs and corporate structures. Being a team player does not necessarily preclude acting with courage. Yet it does diminish the likelihood that individual physicians who are gatekeepers for larger designs and interests will speak out courageously about inequities or on behalf of patients when the necessity arises.

More than physical courage is required to treat patients with dangerous diseases, particularly AIDS. The problem of acting with courage is compounded for today's health professionals by the possible consequences of contracting AIDS. It takes physical and moral courage to run even a very small risk with an invariably terminal future disease. It takes even more fortitude to disclose to patients the fact that one has AIDS. It may mean that one's practice will be curtailed or even closed down, as happened to Dr. Neal Rzepkowski, a physician who volunteered information about his HIV-positive status to administrators and selected patients.[16]

Having the fortitude to face adversity and yet bring about the good is a moral obligation for all human beings. But in today's environment of managed health care, physicians are often seen as providers of services and patients as consumers. It is very easy to shift responsibility. This is true not only for all corporate persons in modern society, even but more so for physicians, who must act in the best interest of their patients.[17] Those interests are at risk of being supplanted by interests like the doctor's own self-interest, those of the hospital, the managed health care system, or society in general.

In Chapter 8 we argued that prudence is at the heart of the medical enterprise precisely because it strengthens clinical and ethical judgment. The same strengthening is represented by fortitude. Fortitude is the kind of tenacity that helps physicians move the powers that be to get their patients into an appropriate clinic for tests. Or it is the tenacity to continue to accept Medicaid payments when they only remotely approximate the costs of caring for the poor. Or it is the courage to speak out strongly in favor of care for all the sick, the poor, the needy; to expose fraud and incompetence; to acknowledge the failings of the current health care system when needed; and to contribute to the public debate about the distribution, availability, and access to health care for all.

Fortitude also played a role in Dr. Rzepkowski's case. Although he voluntarily informed his superiors and in many cases his patients that he had AIDS, no one protested until increasing pressure for disclosure arose when patients apparently contracted AIDS from a dentist in Florida. Even though there is no evidence that physicians have ever infected patients with AIDS, the president of Brooks Memorial Hospital in upstate New York announced Rzepkowski's forced resignation on the basis of such fears. It ended his career at the age of thirty-nine. He was the first health care worker forced to resign, since new guidelines from the Centers for Disease Control in Atlanta initially recommended that physicians with the virus tell patients and refrain from performing invasive procedures.[18] These losses of both professional work and personal status are real possibilities. They have to be faced along with the fear of death from the HIV infection.

It is also a medical virtue not to act rashly or self-righteously to the point of ineffectiveness. The physician cannot expect to change society alone. Enlisting others in the enterprise is important. Among other things, it provides an important check on misguided zealotry. Many physicians are aware of how national policy, say about DRGs, may harm their own patients. But they are uncertain to what extent they are obligated to try to change the system. That task is notoriously difficult. To speak out may brand one as "difficult" or not a "team player." It may compromise a career, cause loss of referrals, or drive patients away. Taking time from the clinical setting, from one's surgical practice, from the examining room, to lobby legislators may not make the most effective use of the power of the physician to bring about good.

Here is where the virtue of prudence discussed in Chapter 8 acts as the guiding virtue. It tells us when courage has exceeded the mean, shading into rashness to its self-defeat.

Medical Fortitude in Society Today

We are now able to define medical fortitude as the virtue that inspires confidence that physicians will resist the temptation to diminish the patient's good through their own fears or through social and bureaucratic pressure, and that they will use their time and training resourcefully to accomplish good in society. There are several characteristics of our society today that make the practice of fortitude very difficult.

First, our society is distressingly callous toward suffering. In part this is a characteristic of mass society often noted by its critics.[19] But in part it stems from the impersonality of the age. We live in a time when treatment is offered not so much by our primary care physician, who might be our friend in the community, but by strangers and specialists whom we must trust to care for us and respect our values. Personal values are difficult to preserve in the depersonalized health care environment of our day. Patients feel estranged from their physicians as a result.

This cuts both ways. Physicians, too, feel estranged from their patients. They live in fear of litigation. They are subject to excessive demands on time and personal life. In addition to these fears are the overwhelming burdens of debt after medical school and professional burnout. Bureaucratic structures of health care encourage dysfunctional behaviors between doctors and society, aggravated by impairments in the primary relationship with patients themselves.[20]

Second, the roots of fortitude are cut off in modern society. We lack the community of values that nurtures the ability to sacrifice present rewards for future ones and to control our present impulses for more satisfying commitments to fundamental values. Thus, not only are physicians estranged from their patients, and also from their patient's values, they must function in an impersonal health care environment in which they meet each other warily as strangers. Fundamental values of the profession itself are questioned by society and by patients. This tends to isolate the physician further from a supporting community. Spirit and the virtues are encapsulated into legalisms. No wonder that today's physician might be tempted to put self-interest first in such an environment. This is so important a problem that we devote later chapters to the virtues of self-effacement and intellectual honesty that are greatly at risk today.

Third, consequently, citizens are easy targets for narcissistic advertising. "Go ahead," we are urged; "reward yourself." "Why not act on impulse? No one else is looking out for you." In this environment, fewer people are willing to run risks. No one wants to be accused of holier-than-thou attitudes or of unrealistic degrees of idealism. Indeed, some ethicists would argue that what we call courage is really hubris, since it endangers self-interest and goes against the major vectors of societal mores. In this view, fortitude is not a virtue but an antivirtue, placing one at considerable risk of social ostracism for no possible benefit. If this were true, anyone wishing to act courageously as we have described it would have to have a double dose of courage just to inaugurate an act.

With fortitude, as with the other virtues we have been discussing in this book, there is a tendency to classify any obligation above the most minimal as supererogatory and therefore not ethically required. Here we confront a major, and fourth, feature of modern society: the fragmentation of the community into a collection of isolated individuals. One response to this isolation is to underline the need for rugged "all-American" individualism and a kind of egoistic autonomy as the basis of society and of ethics. Thinkers like Ayn Rand in philosophy,[21] Robert Nozick in social and political philosophy,[22] and H. Tristram Engelhardt, Jr., in medical ethics[23] have convinced many that the only protection against an impersonal society is heightened self-interest and autonomy. Since social relationships are voluntary and secondary to individual self-interest, the obligations of virtues are voluntary and secondary as well. This is not to say that libertarians and other contemporary moral thinkers are opposed to individuals living a virtuous life. Rather, their analysis of the virtues differs from ours in remarkable ways.

We would respond to libertarian philosophy in two ways. While the virtues are considered excellences (*arete*) of character, they are not by that account impossible to attain. To act out of virtue is not the same as supererogation. All of us are called to live virtuous lives, and we are free to do so by our own choice. In one sense, choosing to be a medical professional underscores this commitment to virtue.

Second, and more to the point of the anticommunitarian views espoused above, the virtues are practiced by individuals immersed in the social and cultural era in which they find themselves. It is ironic and indicative of the degree to which we have eroded the classical conception of a good society that many virtues are today seen as vices. Dr. Rzepkowski functions as an example again. His prudence and courage in informing his superiors and many patients that he had AIDS seems, by modern accounts, at best naive and at worst imprudent.

Conclusion

At this juncture, the argument about the nature of the virtues becomes a metaethical argument about the nature of the ideal society and the place of individual virtues within it. It would be presumptuous to claim that by denying the libertarian construal of society, we would miraculously cease being the *Clockwork Orange* civilization we are fast becoming. Despite significant evidence of the breakdown of Western civilization, sufficient pockets of decency still remain to encourage us to promote the ideals of virtue. This is the only antidote to theories that are inimical to social adhesion and commitment to the common good. As MacIntyre and Hauerwas insist, the virtues cannot thrive without the community that supports what we have termed the "hexis of character."[24,25]

Finally, then, the call to be a courageous physician in modern society is now seen as a far more complex task than speaking out on issues or defending the best interests of patients who have been harmed. At the very least, it requires an additional sophistication about the kind of society that one wishes to build up in face of its sometimes terrifying, "drive-by," murderous reality. In fractious times, the greatest courage is required to commit oneself to others precisely because even loved ones may not understand why one would take the risks involved.

Notes

1. "Fortitude," *Webster's Twentieth Century Unabridged Deluxe Edition* (New York: William Collins Publishers, 1980), p. 722.

2. Plato, *Laws,* I, 630b.

3. Plato, *Statesman,* 308e–309e; *Laws,* I, 630a, 3, 696b.

4. Plato, *Laches,* 190e.

5. See D. S. Hutchinson's treatment of relevant texts on this point in his *The Virtues of Aristotle* (London/New York: Routledge and Kegan Paul, 1986), especially pp. 108ff.

6. Aristotle, *Eudemian Ethics,* 1220a38–1220b20.

7. Ibid., 1220b1.

8. St. Thomas Aquinas, *Summa Theologiae,* Ia2ae, q.60, art. 1. All translations from the Latin are taken from the Blackfriars/McGraw-Hill Book Company edition (New York/London: McGraw-Hill, 1963ff).

9. Aristotle, *Nicomachean Ethics,* Bk. III, c. 7, 1116a10–13.

10. Aquinas, *Summa Theologiae,* 2a2ae, q. 123, a. 9.

11. Ibid., a. 10.

12. Aristotle, *Nicomachean Ethics,* Bk. II, c. 4. 1105a34.

13. Aquinas, *Summa Theologiae,* 2a2ae, q. 123, a. 11.

14. Ibid., a. 11, ad 1.

15. James Drane, *Becoming a Good Doctor: The Place of Virtue and Character in Medical Ethics* (Kansas City, MO: Sheed & Ward/Catholic Health Association, 1988), p. 159.

16. "Doctor with AIDS Virus Forced Out," *Chicago Tribune* (July 28, 1991): Section 1, p. 18.

17. Edmund D. Pellegrino and David C. Thomasma, *For the Patient's Good: The Restoration of Beneficence in Health Care* (New York: Oxford University Press, 1988).

18. See note 16.

19. Lewis Mumford, *The Pentagon of Power: The Myth of the Machine, Vol. 2* (New York: Harcourt Brace & World, 1967–1970).

20. Jurrit Bergsma with David C. Thomasma, *Health Care: Its Psychosocial Dimension* (Pittsburgh: Duquesne University Press, 1983).

21. Ayn Rand, *Atlas Shrugged* (New York: Random House, 1957).

22. Robert Nozick, *Anarchy, State, and Utopia* (Oxford: Basil Blackwell, 1974).

23. H. Tristram Engelhardt, Jr., *The Foundations of Bioethics* (New York: Oxford University Press, 1987).

24. Alasdair MacIntyre, *After Virtue,* 2d ed. (Notre Dame, IN: Notre Dame University Press, 1984).

25. Stanley Hauerwas, *The Community of Character* (Notre Dame, IN: Notre Dame University Press, 1981).

10

Temperance

Given the almost obscene drives encouraged by our modern culture, it is difficult to imagine that any individual, much less a physician, can easily exercise the virtue of temperance. In a society that legitimates conspicuous self-indulgence, the temptations against temperance are many. They range widely, from substance abuse by professionals to the inappropriate use of modern medical technology.

Traditionally, temperance is seen as a virtue that controls one's appetites for food, drink, and sex. But we wish to expand this view to cover some of the more usual temptations of modern professionalism. We do so, as in our other chapters, by first delineating the classical notions of the virtue, then the contemporary extremes that are avoided by cultivating this virtue, and finally, the implications of the virtue for the life of a physician today.

Temperance and Dysfunctional States of Being

The greatest temptations of our modern age are excesses of all sorts. The human appetite has been celebrated for its own sake since the Romantic era in art, music, and architecture. These excesses have been countered by efforts from all quarters to rein in our appetites for environmental and personal destruction. In fact, one could easily argue that movements to temper our use of animals in research, to be environmentally aware, and to moderate our diets by avoiding cholesterol, fat, and salt are all efforts to moderate excessive pampering of the self that is the inheritance of a cultural Romanticism that exalted self-expression in life and profession for its own sake.

Temperance is defined by Plato as a process of doing good in one's business or affairs.[1] Sometimes it is almost synonymous with virtue itself, of doing good, of knowing what we know and do not know, of the health of the soul.[2] It is a kind of modesty about what an individual can and cannot do, knows and does not know. This definition demonstrates how temperate persons might appear boring and repressed in light of our current social values. Contrast this virtue with its opposite, immodesty and arrogance, as displayed, say, by a Madonna video on MTV or by a pampered athletic, scientific, or business genius.

The heart and soul of a virtuous life includes temperance, since this is the way the virtues are brought to bear on the challenges of life itself. Later, when we discuss whether the virtues can be taught, we will reference Plato's famous symbol of the cave, in which individuals see only shadows of reality. It is assumed often that Plato was far more interested in the realities of the Ideas than in the shadowy substances of reality, as symbolized by the cave. Yet for him, training in the moral life included returns from ivory tower contemplation to the realm of experience in the cave:

> . . . you will have to send them [students] down into the cave again, and compel them to hold commands in war and the other offices suitable to youth, that they may not fall short of the other type in experience either. And in these offices, too, they are to be tested to see whether they will remain steadfast under diverse solicitations or whether they will flinch and swerve.[3] Plato, like Aristotle after him, did not think that one could have enough experience to understand the world of Ideas until one was fifty, as a person who "survived the tests and approved themselves altogether the best in every task and form of knowledge."[4]

So temperance, among the important virtues in this task of gaining experience, represents a kind of victory over desire,[5] a science of the self,[6] a self-control that can support the task of being equal to all of life's challenges.[7] In this the individual's self-mastery is equated not only with moderation and modesty, but with wisdom. For this reason, temperance is even called the virtue of the philosopher because the desires "have been taught to flow in the channel of learning. . . . They will be concerned with the pleasures of the soul in itself, and will be indifferent to those of which the body is the instrument."[8]

For Aristotle, temperance also governs bodily pleasures. He defines it thus: "temperance is a mean with regard to pleasures."[9] Aristotle's analysis of the typical human being is filled with wisdom. Such a person craves all the pleasant things in life and, because of this, is led to choose the most pleasant at the cost of everything else. Due to this characteristic of our appetites, it is ironic that there is a loss of equanimity when one does not achieve the pleasure one wants. Aristotle comments drolly about such pleasures: "he is pained both when he fails to get them and when he is merely craving for them (for appetite involves pain); but it seems absurd to be pained for the sake of pleasure."[10]

In keeping with his doctrine about virtue being a mean between two extremes,[11] Aristotle argues that the temperate person avoids insensitivity (even animals know to avoid certain kinds of food, he notes). Temperate persons occupy a "middle position" regarding things that they want, things that they should not want, and any kind of excess.[12] Recall what we said in a previous chapter about virtues being choices that one makes to become a more perfect person. Self-indulgence is also voluntary. So, in a way, intemperance is a voluntary state of soul in which hedonism and a lust for power predominate over wisdom about the body and its needs. It is a childishness of spirit.

It is intriguing to examine how thoroughly St. Thomas treats temperance as the virtue that guides daily human needs like those for food, drink, sex, and companionship towards "intelligent living."[13] The everyday virtues and vices that arise in the treatment of this virtue are many: sobriety, abstinence, gluttony, fasting, drunkenness, chastity, lust, and virginity. But eventually,[14] even more intriguing passions are examined as coming under the purview of temperance: continence in sexual matters, clemency and gentleness, anger and cruelty, modesty and humility, inquisitiveness, good manners, a love of learning, style, and fashion, and pride itself. Aristotle also speaks of magnanimity (greatness of soul) and certain other characteristics of the elite person.[15] That is not our point here. We will focus on pride and the lust for power in our subsequent analysis.

St. Thomas regards temperance, along with the companion virtues of fortitude, prudence, and justice, as "cardinal" virtues, that is, chief or principal virtues in relation to which discussion of other closely related virtues can take place. These virtues themselves are intimately related to one another. If one's character includes a tendency to take command, one might also have other, less noble characteristics: a need for power, hypercriticism, and the like. These must be tempered most of the time, but prudential judgment may require them in certain situations. Sometimes such an individual leads efforts to change society to achieve justice, as did Martin Luther King, with great fortitude and an equally fine sense of prudential judgment. So temperance itself is involved in justice, in fortitude, and in prudential judgment. Another example: reputedly, Toscanini coupled immense powers of concentration and memory in his conducting, but he was seen as almost tyrannical about music-making, putting it before all else. For this good, his intemperance was tolerated. As Harvey Sachs says of this trait:

> By the time he reached adolescence Arturo Toscanini was completely possessed by his love of music and by his desire to get inside it, and the other aspects of his life were of secondary importance. One could call this a distorted point of view; and the distortion was so pronounced in this case that it was eventually to make life difficult for many people who came in direct contact with it, and sometimes insufferable for the man who was its direct victim. But the mental discipline which that distortion demanded also brought its own form of healthiness.[16]

In our day, it is important to emphasize that hedonistic goals occur more often than they might have in the Middle Ages, given the power we have to control our environment, to provide readily for food and drink, fashion, and sexual fulfillment. In fact, it seems today more an explicit goal to indulge oneself than to try to live a more perfect life. Aristotle's theory of happiness has received a lot of criticism. And yet it seems difficult to deny that human good lies in pursuing the excellences that are built into our nature, not the least of which is the control of our passions by reason.[17]

This point brings us back to the argument of Plato that temperance relates directly to living life philosophically, under rational control. Hobbes, for example, held that reason is merely a means to obtain the ends established by human desires, whereas Spinoza held the more classical view that human desires "must be transformed by the ends which rational inquiry sets for rational men."[18] Spinoza lived in a time when other thinkers, like Hobbes, pointed to the obvious restlessness in human nature, the almost mindless pursuit of one desire after the other. But he did not accept this accurate description at face value. Rather, as MacIntyre illustrates:

> He concludes that the supreme good consists in the enjoyment of a human nature which, because it is perfectly aware of its place and its unity with the whole natural scheme of things, accepts the inevitability and necessity of the natural order.[19]

The problem of our day is that the abuse of technology and science lead in the opposite direction, toward altering the natural order and expanding our control over it. Physicians and patients must make moral sense of this kind of power.

"Playing God"

Physicians have always used specialized knowledge for the interests of patients. Controlling this knowledge has given the profession and the individual physician great authority in society, in daily affairs, and within the doctor–patient relationship. Modern medical technology empowers individuals beyond their normal capacities. Because technology is, by definition, an extension of human work, it tempts us to exceed the bounds of temperance. This leads to a kind of paternalism in which individuals comes to believe that they know best what is good for another person by employing the powers technology now invests in these individuals.

Medical technology adds to this traditional paternalism an even greater temptation: the temptation to "play God." Its opposite, a pusillanimous abandonment of patients without sufficient intervention, is found less often, but this may occur when inappropriate judgments about either the patient's values or the patient's quality of life are made.

At the outset, it must be admitted that human beings have an incredible thirst for power. Surely this is one reason that humanity is perpetually dissatisfied with the *status quo* and, therefore, with the restless attempts at change for the better that characterize our progress through history. General Electric Corporation used to have an advertisement that proclaimed: "Progress is our most important product." Progress in what? one might ask. The answer cannot be just technological improvement. To lead a good life, it must include mastery of life's vicissitudes. There is nothing intrinsically wrong with our efforts to improve our lives. On the contrary, it is part of the mission of all human beings to use their facilities and propensities to bring about good in their lives and in society.

Sometimes, however, the lure of mastery of the environment, the circumstances of one's life, the future of civilization overwhelms us. It results not in improvements or empowerments for the better, but rather increased dependency, fear, and an "anxiety of possibilities." One example that foreshadows all others in this century is atomic power and its destructive potential. Indeed, for many, this represents the modern example of the story of human pride and folly told by the Tower of Babel story in the Old Testament. To build the Tower, the human community destroyed itself.

Another example of technology gone amok is that of life-prolonging technology, as discussed earlier. In this regard, Jonsen wonders what exactly life support supports: "We talk about the maintenance of life; we don't often talk about the maintenance of personhood. It interests me little," he says, "indeed, not at all, to be alive as an organism. In such a state I have no interests. It is enormously interesting for me to be a person . . . it is the perpetuation of my personhood that interests me; indeed, it is probably my major and perhaps my sole real interest."[20]

Many technologies developed for specific groups of patients are now used for other patient populations in whom their effect has yet to be evaluated. Because the equipment makes the provider feel better, it is used. When technologies such as dialysis or cardiopulmonary resuscitation become more accessible, there is less of an imperative to justify their use. When ICU beds are plentiful, dying patients are tucked into them.

The effect of overuse of technology without evaluation of its efficacy, and frequently without the patient's consent or even over the patient's objections, is to increase patient and family suffering. It may prolong the suffering of dying, and it creates social suffering by wasting resources that might benefit those with potentially reversible diseases. The ICU is a prime illustration of both the effective use and misuse of technology in our society. The cost of an ICU bed is approximately $2,000 to 3,000 a day.[21] Other hospital beds cost about one-half that amount. From 70 to 80% of patients leave the ICU alive. Many of these are postoperative patients. But of those who are critically ill with chronic disease or major medical or surgical problems, the mortality rate is 40 to 60%. A case in point comes from treatment of AIDS. According to NIH statistics, the mortality rate in ICUs for ventilated AIDS patients is at least 85%. Those with a first incidence of pneumonia often benefit from the ICU. Indeed, the ICU is a major benefit to patients for whom it was designed. But the weak or chronically ill will die almost certainly tethered to their machines in that environment for which it was not designed.[22]

In fact, the problem of euthanasia, as well as the incredibly difficult questions about human reproduction, and all the others in between the origin of life and the final moment of death, involve the question of dominion over life. Because of our technology, the temptation to take control of life itself is almost overwhelming. In health care, more options do not necessarily translate into better health care. Thus, mapping the genome will not only increase our store of knowledge about the complexity of the human genetic structure, but will also lead to genetic therapies and, not too far in the future, to interventions to improve this structure before conception itself.

Cautions about this technology differ from cautions about using the means at our disposal to kill patients at the end of their lives. In the former instance, interventions are worrisome because they appear to redesign nature and life itself. For centuries, however, we have taken the power over life and used it for good or ill. In the latter instance, euthanasia, the worries are somewhat different. Individuals themselves must request it. Nonetheless, even when individuals might request assisted suicide or direct euthanasia, is it not wise to temper the power at our disposal so that we do not inauthentically take on dominion over the lives of others?

By contrast to the perplexing problem of direct euthanasia, inappropriate withdrawal and withholding of care is also a form of "playing God," since it involves one individual, entrusted with the care of another, making judgments about the value of that person's life. It is important to distinguish here between objective evaluation of interventions and outcomes on the well-being of the patient and subjective quality-of-life judgments in which the physician judges that the life the patient is now living is not worthwhile.

For the United States today, the danger exists in the economic sphere.[23] Will it be easier to use a simple method of "dispatching" those persons whose care costs too much, or who are now considered to be a burden on society, like the aged and the poor, than to address their suffering, which sometimes is overwhelming even for the most dedicated caregivers? As Joseph Cardinal Bernardin noted in an address on euthanasia at the University of Chicago Hospital, "We cannot accept a policy that would open the door to euthanasia by creating categories of patients whose lives can be considered of no value merely because they are not conscious."[24] James Bopp, general counsel of the National Right to Life Committee, commenting on the *Cruzan* case, argued that society cannot establish a general rule that third parties can end the lives of persons in permanent vegetative states.[25] While morally valid surrogates who express the intent of the incompetent patient about the care in question may make such decisions, the issue does focus on the importance of maintaining compassionate respect for human life in our society.

This is the real issue for Cardinal Bernardin, for example, who poses this question: "What would we be suggesting to one another and to our society, if, seemingly with the best of motives, we were to say that those who are sick, infirm, or unconscious may be killed? How could we allege that such actions would not affect us individually and collectively"?[26] Such actions are a form of "privatizing life," denying its social and communal dimensions as both a private and a public good.

Therefore, the concerns of disvaluing human life through technical responses to human suffering should not be dismissed as hopelessly conservative and neurotic. The overbearing experience of the twentieth century is one in which persons have been put at the mercy of technology. Caution about this reversal of the creative process, wherein persons are now subject to their own creations, is not only justified but important in developing any social policy and legislative process.

Taking Responsibility for Technology

Medical temperance now can be defined as the constant disposition of physicians toward responsible use of power for the good of their patients, avoiding, on the one hand, underuse of technology and other interventions, with its consequent abandonment of patients, and, on the other, overuse of interventions and technology. The responsible use of power resides in a clinical ethical judgment in every case about the best balance of interventions and outcomes.

This virtue of temperance, perhaps more than any of the others we have discussed, requires of physician an almost exquisite awareness of the physical condition of the patient (to assess outcomes) and the values of patients or their surrogates (to assess the quality of those outcomes measured against the patient's values). This knowledge is essential if a proper balance is to be struck between over- and undertreatment. Another way of expressing the essential quality of temperance is in the term "therapeutic parsimony"—using only those interventions that may result in a reasonable ordering of effectiveness, benefit, and burdens.[27] A physician with the habitual capacity to make this judgment correctly would possess the virtue of temperance.

The most dramatic instances of temperance are culled from the decisions on withholding and withdrawing care from the dying. But temperance is also required to assess properly the interventions to be given to the weak and debilitated elderly, to the demented, to individuals who wish to exercise their autonomy in ways that are easily judged to be self-destructive, and to children, to mention just a few of the challenges.

Dramatic advances have occurred in establishing the rights of patients to determine the treatments they desire or reject, not only during the dying process but also at any time during life. Patient advocacy groups have sponsored and supported legislation, and the courts have largely concurred. In some cases the courts have actively encouraged such legislation, prodding our representatives to develop better legal protections for incompetent patients, surrogates, and the physicians involved in making difficult decisions. The living will, advance directives, and the durable power of attorney are instruments that protect these rights.[28] They will have an impact on long-term care settings,[29] which need further study. What is important to note is that the underlying motivation for the development of such instruments is the protection of the patient's right to live according to his or her deeply held values.[30,31]

But all these measures must aim at temperance—the optimum balance between benefits, effectiveness, and burdens. Thus, absolutization of the patient's autonomy is a subject of growing tension. Concerns about libertarian assumptions implied by this emphasis have led many thinkers to counter autonomy with the need for beneficence as well.[32,33] The implications of conflicts about medical ethics and ethical theory for active euthanasia include the libertarian push for active euthanasia that endangers the health provider's values in caring for the dying patient. This push may diminish the moral quality of the relation between physician and patient. It clearly tends to place exclusive emphasis on the needs and wants of the individual patient. Ultimately, euthanasia raises questions about the kind of society we ought to be.

There is serious concern about the impact on the community when physicians are involved in voluntary active euthanasia.[34] Thus, Leon Kass presents a thoughtful articulation of what is owed a dying patient by the physician. He argues that humanity is owed humanity, not just "humaneness," that is, being merciful by killing the patient. Kass argues that the very reason we are compelled to put animals out of their misery is that they are *not* human and thus demand from us some measure of humaneness. By contrast, human beings demand from us our humanity itself. This thesis, in turn, rests on the relationship "between the healer and the ill" as constituted, essentially, "even if only tacitly, around the desire of both to promote the wholeness of the one who is ailing."[35] This is still a majority view among physicians.

Studies have shown that physicians do not evaluate whether a patient is dying solely on the basis of biomedical data. They also take into account the important features of human interaction, as well as the proportion between therapeutically available interventions and the possible outcome.[36] Such interactive concerns tend to present counterpressures to a straightforward honoring of patients' wishes and autonomy with respect to euthanasia requests. Needless to say, fears about litigation also contribute to reluctance to honor patients' requests even for increases in pain control medication.

The temptation to employ technology rather than to give oneself as a person in the process of healing is a "technological fix." The technological fix is much easier to conceptualize and implement than the more difficult processes of a truly human engagement. The training and skills of modern health professionals overwhelmingly foster the use of technological fixes. By instinct and proclivity, all persons in a modern civilization are tempted by technical rather than personal solutions to problems.

As noted above, medical technology gives us enormous power over all levels of life, but especially at the end of life. Yet concerns should not be confined to "dispatching" persons too early by engaging in active, direct euthanasia while failing to meet their physical and social needs. Another aspect of the "technofix" society is prolonging suffering in conditions of hopeless injury to life. "Hopeless injury" as Braithwaite and Thomasma define it, is

> a condition in which there is no potential for growth or repair; no observable pleasure or happiness from living . . . and a total absence of one or more of the following attributes of quality of life: cognition or recognition, motor activity, memory or awareness of time, consciousness, and language or other intelligent means of communicating thoughts or wishes.[37]

Daily life is full of interactions with things—nonhuman and fundamentally incomprehensible to most persons. We sometimes become so used to technological processes that we behave as though they are substitutes for human and compassionate care. Eating for many elderly and dying patients has been replaced by tubes; participating in the spiritual and material values of human life has been replaced by merely surviving, as "beings" subjugated to the very products of human imagination. As Illich observes:

> Medical civilization is planned and organized to kill pain, to eliminate sickness, and to abolish the need for acts of suffering and dying. . . .[38]

> The new experience that has replaced dignified suffering is artificially prolonged, opaque, depersonalized maintenance.[39]

Such beings on depersonalized maintenance may no longer be as respected as the rest of us precisely because of this subjugation. This is no way to respect the value of human life. Is a permanently unconscious being without any ability to relate to its environment a person? Part of taking responsibility for our technology is to avoid this subjugation of human life to machinery in the first place through more thorough discussions of possible outcomes and patient values regarding them.

Conclusion

In a society such as ours, with its problems of poverty, homelessness, gaining access to health care, and denigration of the weak, we need to maintain constant vigilance about protecting persons from undertreatment, abandonment, and inappropriate overtreatment. In both instances, we will be shepherding our technology to good human aims. This is medical temperance.

Notes

1. Plato, *Charmides*, 161b–e.
2. Ibid., 167a; *Gorgias*, 504c, 507.
3. Plato, *Republic*, VII, 539d–e.
4. Ibid., 540a.
5. Plato, *Phaedrus*, 237e.
6. Plato, *Charmides*, 165d.
7. Plato, *Phaedo*, 68.
8. Plato, *Republic*, VI, 485e.
9. Aristotle, *Nichomachean Ethics*, Bk. III, c. 10, 1117b, 24–25.
10. Ibid., c. 11, 1119a.
11. William F. R. Hardie, *Aristotle's Ethical Theory*, 2d ed. (Oxford: Clarendon Press, 1980), pp. 129–151.
12. Aristotle, *Nichomachean Ethics*, Bk. III, c. 11, 1119a, 10–15.
13. St. Thomas Aquinas, *Summa Theologiae*, 2a2ae, Q.141, a.1.
14. Ibid., QQ. 155–170.
15. Aristotle, *Nichomachean Ethics*, 1123a34–1125a17.
16. Harvey Sachs, *Toscanini* (New York: Harper & Row, Perennial Library, 1988), p. 12.
17. D.S. Hutchinson, *The Virtues of Aristotle* (New York: Routledge and Kegan Paul, 1986), p. 39.
18. Alasdair MacIntyre, "Spinoza," *Encyclopedia of Philosophy*, Vol. 7–8, ed. Paul Edwards (New York: Macmillan and the Free Press, 1967), p. 540.
19. Ibid., p. 531.
20. Albert R. Jonsen, "What Does Life Support Support?" *Personal Choices and Public Commitments: Perspectives on the Humanities*, ed. W. Winslade, (Galveston, TX: Institute for the Medical Humanities, 1988), pp. 66–67.
21. Thomas A. Raffin, Joel N. Shurkin, and Wharton W. Sinkler, *Intensive Care: Facing the Critical Issues* (New York: W.H. Freeman, 1988), p. 185.
22. Ibid., p. 175.
23. Ann A. Scitovsky and Alexander M. Capron, "Medical Care at the End of Life: The Interaction of Economics and Ethics," *Annual Review of Public Health Reports* 7 (1986):59–75.
24. J. Bernardin, *Euthanasia: Ethical and Legal Challenge: Address to the Center for Clinical Medical Ethics*, University of Chicago Hospital, May 26, 1988. Unpublished manuscript, p. 16.
25. M. Weinstein, "United States Supreme Court to Hear First Case Involving Right-to-Die," *American College of Physicians Observer* (9) (July–August 1989):9.
26. Bernardin, *Address*, p. 14.
27. Edmund D. Pellegrino and David C. Thomasma, *For the Patient's Good: Toward the Restoration of Beneficence in Health Care* (New York: Oxford University Press, 1989).
28. Chris Hackler, Ray Moseley, and Dorothy E. Vawter (eds.), *Advance Directives in Medicine* (New York: Praeger, 1989).

29. F. Rouse, "Living Wills in the Long-Term Care Setting," *Journal of Long-Term Care Administration* (17) (Summer 1988):14–19.

30. A. Mehling, "Living Wills: Preventing Suffering or a Deadly Contract?" *State Government News* (December 1988):14–15.

31. A. Mehling and S. Neitlich, "Right-to-Die Backgrounder," *News from the Society for the Right to Die,* January 1989. Newsletter of 4 pages.

32. Pellegrino and Thomasma, *For the Patient's Good.*

33. Erich Loewy, "The Restoration of Beneficence," *The Hastings Center Report* 19 (1989):42–43.

34. W. Gaylin, L. Kass, E. D. Pellegrino, and M. Siegler, "Commentaries: Doctors Must Not Kill," *Journal of the American Medical Association* 259(14) (April 8, 1988):2139–2140.

35. L. Kass, "Arguments Against Active Euthanasia by Doctors Found at Medicine's Core," *Kennedy Institute of Ethics Newsletter* 3 (January 1989):1–3, 6.

36. J. Muller and B. Koenig, "On the Boundary of Life and Death: The Definition of Dying by Medical Residents," *Biomedicine Examined,* ed. M. Lock and D. Gordon (Dordrecht/Boston: Kluwer, 1988), pp. 351–374.

37. S. Braithwaite, and D. C. Thomasma, "New Guidelines on Foregoing Life-Sustaining Treatment in Incompetent Patients: An Anti-Cruelty Policy," *Annals of Internal Medicine* 104 (1986):711–715.

38. Ivan Illich, *Medical Nemesis: The Expropriation of Health* (New York: Pantheon Books, 1976), p. 106.

39. Ibid., p. 154.

11

Integrity

Integrity without knowledge is weak and useless, and knowledge without integrity is dangerous and dreadful.

SAMUEL JOHNSON, *Rasselas*, 1759

This chapter will examine the virtue of integrity and its subsidiary, intellectual honesty, in light of the many dangers of compromise that occur, especially in biomedical research. Integrity, by its very connotation, defines for us the nature of the individual who integrates all of the virtues. To say that someone possesses integrity is to claim that that person is almost predictable about responses to specific situations, that he or she can integrate all the virtues into a whole and can prudentially judge the relative importance in each situation of principles, rules, guidelines, precepts, and the other virtues in reaching a decision to act. Clearly, a virtuous physician and a virtuous patient, working in a concert of interests that is the doctor–patient relationship, must possess this virtue to bring about the healing aim of the relationship.

The Virtue of Integrity in Clinical Practice

Despite the dominance of autonomy thinking in recent biomedical ethics, integrity is the more fundamental concept. The moral claim to autonomy rests on the deeper moral claim of all humans to integrity of the person. In the first part of this chapter, we examine autonomy and integrity in the physician–patient relationship and their moral implications for both parties. We include the relationship of autonomy and integrity to trust, without which neither of the two concepts can realistically be actualized. Because we have already sketched the virtue of trust, this interrelationship is discussed only briefly here.

Autonomy—the Legal and Moral Concepts

In the last twenty-five years, autonomy has emerged as the dominant notion in biomedical ethics in America and increasingly in the rest of the world. This is a sharp departure from the tradition of benign paternalism that characterized the

Hippocratic tradition for 2,500 years. The impetus for this shift in the locus of decision has been sociopolitical and philosophical.

The sociopolitical forces behind the emergence of autonomy need only be enumerated for our purposes here. They derive from a convergence of many forces: the progressive spread of participatory democracy, a mistrust of authority and technical expertise, the expansion of public education, the intrusions of law and economics into medical ethics, and the necessity to confront the challenges of technology in a morally pluralistic society. Together, these forces engendered mistrust of the physician and a demand for greater participation in medical decisions. As a result, autonomy has become a watchword symbolizing the moral and legal claim of patients to make their own decisions without constraint or coercion by physicians, however beneficent their intentions may be.

Legally, the principle of autonomy derives from the right to privacy. This right is not explicitly stated in the U.S. Constitution but has been derived in a series of Supreme Court decisions as a penumbra of the Bill of Rights. The American concept of a "right to privacy" in one's home and personal life has a long and complicated history.[1] The right to privacy now extends to cover rights to decide on the education of children, choice of marriage partner, religious preference, access to contraceptive devices, and termination of pregnancy.[2] In 1914 this right to privacy was extended specifically to include the right to reject lifesaving medical treatments.[3] This right of refusal has in the last two decades been progressively extended to include withdrawal of life support measures, first in terminally ill patients and then in nonterminal patients, from those with total to those with partial brain death, and from competent patients to patients' surrogate or their wishes expressed in a living will or medical directive.[4] Today the right to privacy is the dominant legal restraint on the traditional paternalism of physicians.

Morally, the principle of autonomy has several sources. One is Locke's *Second Treatise on Government,* which held men in the state of nature to be free and equal, so that none might have sovereignty over another except through a social contract freely entered into.[5] Locke's arguments gave rise to the notion of "negative rights"—rights not to be interfered with by others. These negative rights have come to be the foundation of liberal democracy for many people.

A second powerful and influential philosophical moral claim to autonomy is propounded in Kant's *Groundwork for a Metaphysics of Morals.*[6] Here Kant argues that freedom is essential to all morality, that it is identical with autonomy, and that autonomy is "the ground of the dignity of human nature and of every rational nature."[7] Kant unites the idea of a rational being with dignity this way: "a rational being himself must be the ground for all maxims of action never merely as a means, but as a supreme condition restricting the use of every means, that is, always also as an end."[8] The dignity of man "consists precisely in his capacity to make universal law, although only on condition of being himself subject to the law he makes."[9]

A third source for a moral claim to autonomy is John Stuart Mill's essay "On Liberty." Mill asserts that the only restraint on liberty is harm to others, not harm to self. It is this latter notion, joined with the Lockean idea of negative rights, that seems to be the connecting link between the philosophical notion of autonomy and the legal notion of privacy most influential with the courts in America. This is the principle generally used to resolve conflicts about who should make the final decision on accepting or rejecting medical treatments. This seems to be the case with the reports of the President's commission as well.[10]

The conjunction of the legal conception of privacy and the moral concept of autonomy has crystallized into a widely accepted medical decision-making paradigm. Competent patients have the moral and legal claim to make their own decisions, and these decisions take precedence over those of the doctor or the family. When patients are no longer competent (or have never been competent, such as, infants or the retarded), their right to make decisions is transferred to a valid surrogate or to some anticipatory statement, such as a living will, medical directive, or durable power of attorney—or, in the absence of these, to a legally appointed guardian.[11] Some have so absolutized the principle of autonomy and the right of privacy that they would place no limits on its exercise. Others accept varying limits on autonomy. We shall return to these exceptions later when we examine the links between autonomy and integrity.

The most concrete actualization of the principles of privacy and autonomy lies in the doctrine of informed consent, which has become the central requirement of morally valid medical decision-making.[12] For consent to fulfill the claims of human beings to self-governance, it must be based on sufficient information to make a reasoned choice and must be free of coercion or deception. The procedures surrounding informed consent are designed to facilitate the capacity of rational beings to make judgments of what they consider best, rather than what the physician or any other person might consider best for them.

Integrity of Persons and Persons of Integrity

Integrity is a more complex and fundamental notion than autonomy. Etymologically, it means completeness, wholeness, and unity. It has two senses of significance for medical ethics. One sense refers to the integrity of the person, of the patient, and of the physician; the other refers to being a person of integrity. In the first sense, integrity is a moral claim that belongs to every human simply by virtue of being human. In the second sense, integrity is a virtue, moral soundness and wholeness. It is a moral habitus acquired by its constant practice in our relation with others. Each sense of integrity has important ethical implications in medical ethics.

Integrity of the person. By the integrity of the person, we mean the right ordering of the parts in relation to the whole, the balance and harmony between the various dimensions of human existence necessary for the healthy functioning of the whole organism. The integrity of persons is expressed in a balanced relationship between the bodily, psychosocial, and intellectual elements of their lives. No one element is out of proportion to the others. Each takes the lead when the good of the whole requires it. Each stands ready to yield to the others in the interests of the whole. Integrity in this sense is synonymous with health.

In this view, illness and disease are forms of dis-integration, of dis-unity of the person in which overall functioning is impeded. With physical illness, the body usurps the central role and becomes the focus of attention, rather than the means to the pursuit of work, play, or human relationships. Similarly, psychological illness is a form of dis-integration in which anxieties, obsessions, and illusions assume controlling positions, distorting the balance and unity of a person's life.

Illness also assaults the unity of the self and its relationship with the body. Ordinarily, body and self are in close unity. When illness afflicts us, we feel alienated from the afflicted part. We stand away from the body, reject it, or resent it. The sick body or mind rebels against the whole. The self itself becomes fractured. The image we have fashioned of our identity is threatened by illness. We each live with a unique balance we have struck over the years between our hopes and aspirations and the limitations imposed by our physiological, psychological, or physical short-comings. Serious illness forces a confrontation with the impact of disability, pain, and death on that image. These require the restructuring of a new image with new points of balance and a new definition of what constitutes health.

Another facet of integrity of the person is the integrity of the values we cherish and espouse. Each of us in a real sense defined by the particular configuration of values we have chosen as our own. In illness these values may be in conflict with those of the physician, our families, or society. Our conception of healing reflects our assessment of what constitutes good functioning. To be cured or treated, our most cherished values must become the subject of the physician's scrutiny and possible manipulation. The values, thus, are at risk of challenge or damage in the medical transaction.

These two perspectives on integrity of the person and the potential for dis-integration by illness create moral obligations for the physician who purports to heal and help, as well as for the patient. Healing means to make whole again, that is, to reestablish the wholeness that constitutes a healthy existence. This is the aim of medical care and is a covenant inherent in the medical relationship. To be faithful to that covenant, the physician is obliged to remedy the dis-integration of the person inflicted by disease. This includes the psychosocial as well as the physical realm. Restoration of the integrity of the person is the moral basis of any genuinely holistic medicine.

Equally important is the obligation to preserve the integrity of the self and the values that identify the person as a unique individual. It is this vulnerability of the patient's values that generates the obligation to enhance and restore the patient's autonomous capacity for decision making. Autonomy thus is grounded ultimately in the fact that to usurp the patient's human capacity for self-governance is to violate the integrity of her person. To ignore, override, repudiate, or ridicule the patient's values is to assault the patient's very humanity. This aggravates the dis-integration of the person that already exists as a result of illness. Nothing could be further from a morally defensible healing relationship.

The patient's moral claim to respect for her autonomy is not absolute, however. It is limited by the equivalent claim of the physician as a person to his own autonomy. The patient cannot violate the physician's integrity as a person. If the physician is morally opposed to abortion, euthanasia, withdrawal or withholding of food or fluid, or artificial insemination, for example, he cannot be expected to respect the patient's autonomy over his own. This will become an increasingly important matter as morally debatable procedures become legal and parts of a health insurance benefit package. Both physician and patient are entitled to respect for the integrity of their persons; neither may impose his or her values on the other. Respectful withdrawal from the relationship may be necessary to avoid cooperation in acts that might compromise the moral integrity of either the physician or the patient.

Another limitation occurs when a patient's autonomous decision might produce a serious, definable, and direct harm to another person. An example here is the patient who is HIV positive and refuses to have that fact revealed to his spouse or sexual partner. In this instance the physician cannot withdraw. He has the obligation in justice to tell the person at risk after first offering the patient the opportunity to reveal the fact personally.

The autonomous decision of a valid surrogate must also be resisted if there is clear evidence of a conflict of interest, which might lead to the over- or under-treatment of an incompetent adult or infant. The physician's primary obligation is to preserve the integrity of the person of the patient. Under circumstances like these, the physician cannot withdraw but must take the measures available in a democratic society to protect the patient's interests. This may mean reference to an ethics committee, appointment of a legal guardian, or direct court intervention to limit the autonomy of the surrogates.

Indeed, carried to extremes, the morally justifiable claim to autonomy can end by destroying any notion of the communality of human existence. Autonomy absolutized leads to moral atomism, privatism, and anarchy. Humans are social animals. They cannot be fulfilled except in social relationships, as Aristotle so wisely pointed out. The community within which the patient resides has moral claims as well. This communitarian dimension of biomedical ethics is in serious danger of compromise in the current drive for autonomy as the guiding principle of medical ethics.

Patients owe a debt to the community for the lifelong benefits they derive from social relationships. They should feel some duty to limit their demands for expensive or marginally beneficial treatments and technologies that impose financial burdens on society and their families. Voluntary limitations should be placed on life support measures that are futile or that merely prolong the act of dying, out of a sense of social justice.

The moral claim to autonomy, here defined as the capacity of humans to make self-determining choices based on their rational nature, derives from the more fundamental claim for preservation of the integrity of the person. This is a powerful moral claim, and it generates a corresponding duty on the part of other humans to respect it. Yet the claim in medical as well as other human transactions is not absolute. It must be balanced against the equivalent claims of physicians, of other persons, and of justice.

Finally, if we look at autonomy as a derivative of the integrity of the person and not as an isolated ethical principle, the presumed conflict between autonomy and beneficence should disappear. Paternalism cannot be equated with beneficence, as some authors propose. Paternalism involves the physician's usurpation of the patient's moral claim as a human being to decide what is in his or her own best interests. This violates the integrity of the person and under no circumstances could be a beneficent act. Rather, to be beneficent, respect for the patient's values and choices is essential. As we have pointed out elsewhere, the physician holds **beneficence in trust**.[13]

The person of integrity. The law of privacy and the principle of autonomy are necessary but not sufficient to preserve the integrity of the sick person in the medical transaction. What is indispensable is the person of integrity, the person of moral wholeness, who can be trusted to respect the nuances and subtleties of the moral claim to autonomy. The physician, therefore, must be a person who exhibits the virtue of integrity, the person who not only accepts respect for the autonomy of others as a principle but interprets its application in the most morally sensitive way.

The ultimate safeguard of the integrity of the patient's person is the fidelity of the physician to the fiduciary nature of **the healing relationship**. It is the physician who interprets and applies the principle of autonomy. Everything depends upon how the physician presents the facts, which facts she selects and emphasizes, how much and how little she reveals, how she weighs risks and benefits, how she respects or exploits the fears and anxieties of the patient—in sum, how she uses her Aesculpaean power. Every patient, even the most educated and the most independent, becomes a victim or a beneficiary of that power. The resultant responsibility is heavy on the physician to be aware of the dependent, vulnerable, and frightened state of the patient, and not to exploit that state even if she thinks it is in the patient's best interests.

Clearly, no contract, law, or abstract ethical principle can eradicate the need for trust, just as it cannot be eradicated from all other human relationships. The present emphasis on autonomy has been extremely significant in reducing the grosser violations of the integrity of persons. But the physician's responsibility for safeguarding the patient's autonomous wishes still depends strongly on his character.

The physician is the pathway through which decisions, actions, and policies relating to the patient must pass. He is in a position to enhance the patient's self-determination and to block incursions by others. This sensitive position does not give him privileges but only heightened responsibilities to be the guardian of the integrity of the person, of the patient he has a covenant to serve. In this position the physician also becomes the moral accomplice of decisions and policies that may affect the patient's integrity as a person.

Clearly, the physician must be a person of integrity if the integrity of the person is to be safeguarded and healed when it is dis-integrated by illness. At the foundation of medical ethics is the fiduciary relationship and the virtue of fidelity to trust. These dispose the physician to comprehend the meaning of the integrity of the person, and this meaning, in turn, is what grounds the law of privacy and the principle of autonomy.

It must not be forgotten that part of respect for the patient's autonomy and the integrity of the patient's person is the moral right to yield up the right of autonomy itself. Therefore, when the physician has made an honest effort to stimulate the participation of the patient but the patient feels overwhelmed and unable to decide, the patient may ask the physician what should be done. Under these conditions, and only under these conditions, the physician has a moral mandate to make the decision for the patient. Not to do so is a form of moral abandonment.

Under all ordinary circumstances, however, the formula for the most morally reassuring decision-making seems to be this: the decision should not be made by the physician for the patient, nor should it optimally be made by the patient in isolation from the doctor, even if this is phenomenologically possible. Rather, the decision should involve both doctor and patient in a true consensus in which the integrity of each person is protected. The physician should think of making a decision *for* and *with* the patient, "for" signifying not in place of the patient but in the interests of the patient.

We now turn to the importance of integrity in scientific research.

The Virtue of Integrity in Scientific Research

In 1785, in a letter to his nephew Peter Carr, Jefferson wrote: "An honest heart being the first blessing, a knowing head is the second."[14] With his customary concise eloquence, Jefferson strikes the keynote we sound in this section: intelligence is not enough. Character and virtue must precede it in human affairs.

We know the truth of this statement in science. It rests on the ineradicable fact that in the laboratory and at the bedside, when no one is watching, it is the character of the investigator that determines the moral quality of research. If research integrity is problematic, we must start and end with the investigator. Aberrations in the structure of the research system may explain but do not excuse scientific misconduct. It is the misconduct of individual scientists that leads Congress and the public to ask, "Can scientists (not science) be trusted any longer to govern themselves?"

The pertinence of this question was recognized clearly in one of the earliest papers on ethics in clinical research written in 1966. Henry Beecher, after emphasizing the importance of informed consent as a safeguard for the experimental subject concluded: *"there is the more reliable safeguard provided by the presence of an intelligent, informed conscientious, compassionate, responsible investigator."*[15]

Beecher's words succinctly define the character traits of the morally responsible investigator and the locus of accountability for misconduct. Beecher's perspective differs sharply from the responses of some prominent spokesmen of science who insist that the problem is *"not moral but political,"* *"grossly exaggerated,"*[16] or that it is the "ideology" of science, the system of rewards, or the social structure of science that is at fault.[17-19] Here we expand on Beecher's focus on the investigator's character.

Character is the foundation of the moral life. This idea, after years of neglect, is being resuscitated by contemporary ethicists. It has yet to be influential in biomedical ethics, however, where rules, principles, and guidelines have dominated for the last quarter of a century. What we argue here is that an ethic of virtue must complement the existing ethic of principles if we are to have a comprehensive perspective on the ethical behavior of the scientist.

In the interests of clarity, we start with several disclaimers. First, there are many kinds and degrees of scientific misconduct, not all equally grave or morally culpable. We must distinguish between fraud and honest error, between conflict of interest and fraud, and between "cooking," "fudging," or falsifying data. There are thereby different degrees of moral culpability, but sooner or later, all depend upon the character of the investigator.

Second, despite recent disclosures, we do not think that we are in the midst of an epidemic of moral turpitude among scientists. While most scientists are honorable people doing their jobs well, scientific misconduct has been with us for a long time. We do not know its actual incidence or prevalence. If we scan the six-and-a-half pages of "known and suspected cases" since ancient times compiled by Broad and Wade, we are struck by its relative rarity.[20] But its rarity cannot justify trivializing or ignoring fraud, as some apologists of science have suggested.

Third, fraud cannot be viewed solely as the product of "unhinged" or "deranged" minds or the exaggeration of the spectacle-hungry media, as some would aver.[21,22] Likewise, we cannot subscribe to the contention that the scientific community is automatically self-correcting. Nothing invites external regulation more surely than denial of wrongdoing or failure to admit accountability and to take constructive steps for improvement.

Finally, recall that our emphasis on an ethic of virtue and character is not a repudiation of principle- and rule-based ethics, as exemplified in the Nuremburg Code, the Declaration of Helsinki, or the Guidelines for Research Involving Human Subjects prepared by the Council for International Organizations of Medical Science and the World Health Organization.[23–25] The conceptual challenge in biomedical ethics, as in general ethics, is to link principle-based and virtue-based ethics in a mutually reinforcing relationship—not to supplant one with the other.

The Nature of Virtue Ethics in Research

The aim of ethics from its beginnings has been twofold: to teach how to form good character and how to make morally good decisions. For the greater part of the history of ethics, character and virtue were the major foci. Only in recent years has attention switched to making decisions and solving dilemmas in accordance with certain *prima facie* principles.[26] Today, however, the limitations of principle-based ethics are becoming better appreciated. As a result, we are entering an era of renewed interest in virtue both in general and in professional ethics. MacIntyre has ably described the evolution and devolution of virtue ethics and the need for its resuscitation.[27,28]

This is not the place to discuss virtue and character in the larger moral sense of the traits that would make the research scientist a good human being. In our morally pluralistic world, there is distressingly little agreement on what it means to be a good person. What are vices for some are virtues for others. While we are convinced that there are certain character traits or virtues that define a good person, this point will not be argued here. Rather, we are concerned with the virtues or traits of character that enable us to do our work well, that is, to be good researchers, physicians, lawyers, or scientists. MacIntyre has expanded the Aristotelian idea of virtues, discussed in Chapter 1, to define virtues as acquired traits that are necessary to attaining the goods *internal* to a practice.[29] The goods internal to a practice are recognizable in terms of the aims of that practice and the understandings of its practitioner. For example, the good internal to medicine is healing or health, and the virtues of the physician are those traits we need to attain those goods or to overcome the obstacles that frustrate them. MacIntyre also recognizes an important communal dimension in the virtues, since they are learned in, shared with, and necessary for the good of communities.[30] Let us now examine this notion of the virtues with respect to the practice of scientific and medical research.

The good internal to the practice of research is truth, an understanding of what is *really real* about some aspect of the world we inhabit. The virtues of the scientist are those that enable the scientist to attain truth, which is the aim of research. They are the virtues of objectivity, critical thinking, honesty in recording and reporting data, freedom from bias, and sharing of knowledge with the scientific community.

In addition, there is the virtue of fidelity to trust. The public provides funds, facilities, and the conditions conducive to free inquiry in the expectation that they will be used to expand human knowledge for the benefit of all. Those who accept funds for research enter into a covenant with society in which the primary goods cannot be power, personal profit, prestige, or pride. These are secondary goods external to research. They are attainable in other pursuits. They are not specific to the purposes of research. Invariably at the foundation of scientific fraud is an inversion of values and dispositions, so that self-interest replaces truth as the ordering principle. In a word, the goods *external* to the practice dominate and frustrate the attainment of the goods *internal* to the practice.

The Industrial Model of Research

Were this an ideal world and were scientists free of normal human drives, we could end our discussion here. We would need only to define the moral nature of the quest for knowledge and the character traits it entails, and they would be automatically exhibited by every scientist. This is what Plato might have expected, since he equated excellence of character (*arete*) with knowledge of the truth. Vice for Plato was simply ignorance of moral truth. Aristotle was more realistic. He knew by experience, as we do, that humans are creatures of both reason and affect. To know what is good does not guarantee the motivation to do good.

To be sure, we must know the good first. That is why we have emphasized the kind of person the scientist must be if he or she is to be ethical. To remain virtuous, the scientist must cope with a series of challenges inherent in the complex fiscal, professional, and social structure of contemporary scientific research. These challenges all conduce to the vice of *selfish* self-interest. At every turn, there are inducements to self-interest that subvert the purposes of research and violate the public trust.

Self-interest is a normal human motive and is not in itself morally wrong. Aristotle has an extended analysis of the distinction between licit and illicit self-interest that is pertinent to this discussion.[31] Like other human beings, researchers have legitimate self-interests. They seek to advance their careers, provide for their families, and enjoy the approval of their peers and the gratification of honors, public recognition, and leisure. But as Aristotle emphasizes, when these motives dominate and interfere with the ends proper to living an ethically good life or achieving the aims of one's work, they become the wrong kind of self-interest—the vice central to most scientific fraud. "Selfish" self-interest leads to various forms of compromise dangerous to the research subject, the public, and the enterprise of science itself.

The most serious inducements to selfish self-interest arise from the recent metamorphosis of research from a scholarly to an industrial activity. The values of scholarship—seeking truth, reporting honestly, sharing information, restraining bias, and protecting the freedom to choose research subjects—are brought into conflict with the values of industry, commerce, and business. Gaining the competitive edge, establishing priority and ownership of information, cornering the market, getting the patent, choosing research topics on their future investment possibilities—these are the values of industry. They encourage the wrong kind of self-interest and frustrate the primary aim of research.

The industrial model makes research a commodity like any other, an item produced for its exchange value, for what it yields in promotion, tenure, lighter teaching loads, a larger laboratory, more support dollars, and so on. The senior investigator becomes an entrepreneur and a corporate executive whose success is measured in the number of works published, grants received, committee memberships, prizes and the like. Like successful executives, successful scientists are lured from one institution to another by promises of more of everything—from zero teaching loads to stock options.

The industrial model is self-replicating. Young investigators, like yuppie corporate types, mimic their elders, learn to compromise values, and legitimate their climb up the corporate research ladder. The values of the research community become so distorted that what were vices, like secrecy and selective reporting of data, now become virtues. Senior investigators claim credit for even the most tangential contact with a research project but shun responsibility for errors in their laboratories. Moral accountability in the large research team is so diffuse that everyone points to someone else as the culprit when misconduct is discovered.

This distortion of values evokes an understandable response from the public. Science comes to be treated as the industry it tries to be. The public is the consumer of its products. We begin to hear talk of product liability when research is not definitive, magical cures do not result, or data must be reevaluated. Incompetence, fraud, and profit motives are alleged or the investigator gets a "Golden Fleece Award." Scientists and legislators become antagonists. The legislator organizes investigations and elaborates regulations to limit the investigator's freedom.[32] Scientists and the scientific community deny and stonewall, while the public calls for ever more rigorous regulation. Dilution of the scholarly model by the values of industry erodes the intellectual integrity of the research endeavor and distorts the relationship between science and the public.

Note that the academic and scholarly models are not free of the seductions of selfish self-interest. Pride, prestige, and honors are as tempting to some as dollars. The pursuit of profit and the pedant's pursuit of immortality in the citation index can be equally destructive of the ethics of research. But when money and the corporate value system invade science, the normal human pull of self-interest is magnified many times over.

"Selfish" self-interest corrodes the search for truth in every branch of science, but it is particularly dangerous when human subjects are involved. So much has been written on this subject that we will limit our discussion to the abuses most closely linked to the industrialization and commercialization of biomedical research.[33]

Pharmaceutical companies are understandably eager for clinical trials conducted by prestigious investigations and institutions. To this end, they offer a variety of financial incentives. They may furnish part of the investigator's salary, provide certain fringe benefits like travel and accommodations at deluxe resorts for "research" meetings, offer consulting fees, give gifts of various kinds, or offer a share in the profits from the products being tested.

Inducements to self-interest can involve the whole institution. Long-term contractual arrangements between industry and universities are now in vogue. A drug company will support research facilities and personnel in return for privileged access and a share in the patenting rights to the products developed. Industry–university compacts are especially seductive when other sources of research funding are insufficient. These may well turn out to be Faustian compacts. Eventually, universities may have to sacrifice scientific integrity or abrogate their "most favored investigator" status. If corporate profits fall or the "investment" in research is insufficiently productive, industry will take the initiative to reduce its commitment. In either case, the scientific research effort will suffer serious setbacks.

Sharing research data is a traditional practice among scholars. University—industry contracts usually recognize the investigator's right to publish in peer-reviewed journals. But it is a fact of business that one does not alert one's competitors to a new product before it is marketed. It is not unfair to suppose that investigators, for fear of losing long-term research support, might consciously or unconsciously withhold information about a commercially promising discovery.

These potential conflicts of interest pose serious dangers to experimental subjects. They can subtly compromise the process of informed consent, the cornerstone of clinical research ethics.[34,35] They can also compromise beneficence, the central value in medical ethics, as well as truth, the principal value of science. The objectivity, accuracy, and reliability of observations and data interpretation that science requires can subtly be undermined by financial incentives, as well as by institutional and personal pride. Scientific probity and subject safety are the vulnerable victims of self-interest.

The ubiquity, urgency, and complexity of these changes in the structure of research that follow its industrialization are serious threats to the integrity of the investigator. They help to explain why it is more difficult today to be a virtuous investigator. They may even soften our judgments of a particular investigator's culpability. But ethical misconduct is not excusable simply because exigency forces it upon us. Indeed, the difficulties make it even more compelling morally to do whatever we can to prevent scientific misconduct.

Enhancing Ethical Research Behavior

The final safeguard of the moral quality of research is the character and conscience of the investigator, to be sure. But what can we do about it? We can choose between external regulation and legal standards for research, or we can work for internal reforms. If external regulation is to be minimized, it will only be by convincing evidence of internal moral reform. What directions might internal reforms take?

Virtue ethics is concerned with two things: (1) the acquisition by its practitioners of a set of virtues essential to attaining the goods internal to a practice and (2) providing a community of practitioners within which those virtues can be sustained and nourished. Both are theoretically teachable by the study of ethics. Despite the rapid growth of biomedical ethics in the medical curriculum, there has been no parallel development in the sciences *per se*. Immediately, skeptics will ask, can ethics be taught? Is it not too late even in graduate school? Will courses in ethics make people more virtuous? Whose ethics do we teach? The answers to these questions are explored in our penultimate chapter. A solid basis has been established in teaching ethics in medical school curricula.[36,37] We summarize here some suggestions from our experience with medical curricula.

To be effective, teaching ethics to scientists should be done in a regular course and not left to each mentor or instructor. It is an attractive idea for each instructor to integrate the ethical issues relevant to her subject. Experience shows, however, that this method is too uncertain to be relied upon. What is everybody's responsibility ends up being no one's. Most scientists, in any case, do not possess the skills or interests requisite for teaching ethics as a discipline. A separate course, cotaught by a basic scientist and a qualified philosopher-ethicist, is far more likely to be successful.

Teaching must be relevant to science and not limited to an abstract presentation of philosophical principles. The case method, as in medical school teaching of ethics, will be most successful. Concrete cases of scientific misconduct, taken from the history of science and from the contemporary scene, should be analyzed and studied in depth. Principles will emerge from cases, especially if teaching is done in seminar and tutorial fashion, with emphasis on student involvement. This is even more achievable in graduate school, where classes are smaller than in medical schools.

Will courses in ethics do any good? When this question is asked, what most people want to know is whether we can effect changes in behavior or whether we can teach character and virtue. Our answer is a qualified yes. First of all, a course in research ethics should raise ethical sensitivities and should enable students to identify ethical issues, to reflect on their own moral values, to know themselves better, and to better understand the values of others. These effects predispose the student to virtuous conduct, though they do not guarantee it.

The most effective way to teach virtue ethics is through the example of a respected scientist, one whom the student wishes to emulate. This is the way research ethics has been transmitted in the past, and it is not to be denigrated. Unfortunately, too many senior scientists lack ability or interest in teaching ethics, are antipathetic to it as a discipline, or have themselves already compromised the integrity of research standards and are disqualified as models. When good models are not available, character also can be taught from paradigm cases and by the study of the lives and intellectual biographies of ethically admirable scientists, past and present.

Finally, we must remember that virtues are acquired by practice, as both Aristotle and Aquinas insisted. By observing others, by being critical of our own moral choices, and by behaving as a good person would, we learn virtue over the years. The more we practice virtues, the more we perfect our sense of what is and what is not morally acceptable.

What about the established scientist? Must we wait for a new generation before moral reform is a reality? While it is daunting to suggest teaching ethics to senior investigators, there are ways to do so without offending their pride. Again, experiences gained in medicine indicate that education in ethics for practicing physicians is well received if presented in one- or two-day conferences, in intensive courses, or by periodic ethical rounds. Like other teaching sessions, it must be based on case discussions.

Also, we must not underestimate the subtle influence of students taking courses in ethics. They will raise pertinent questions in their other classes and laboratories, forcing even reluctant instructors to take some note of ethical issues. Additional reinforcing measures are journal clubs, visiting lectures, and service on institutional review boards. Editors of scientific journals, worried about the ethics of research and authorship, can do much to stimulate and disseminate ethical discourse among scientists by publishing scholarly papers on ethics, as the best clinical journals already do.

As with medical faculties, there will be obstacles to overcome in science faculties. One is the positivist stance of many scientists, who discount any conclusion or knowledge not susceptible to experimental verification. They discount ethics as mere opinion and ethical discourse as an exercise in futility. This objection is difficult to overcome except by patient and competent discussions that raise concrete issues and emphasize that, like it or not, we do make moral choices. This being the case, we can argue that it is important to be as rigorous in our thinking about ethics as about our experiments.

The other obstacles are the time commitment and evaluation of effectiveness. These are weak objections. The time required is, comparatively, not very great, considering the urgency of the topic and the time given to other topics, often repetitively presented. Evaluation of learning is easy so far as the techniques of ethical analysis are concerned. It is difficult, as indicated above, with respect to changes in character.

By these measures, a gradual understanding of the moral accountability of individual scientists and the centrality of character in scientific integrity will suffuse the whole scientific community. In this way too, the shared values and beliefs of the community necessary to a virtue ethic will be built up. These values will, in turn, serve to sustain the virtues essential to the practice of good science. As the common understanding of character and virtue expands, it will stimulate collective efforts like the elaboration of policies to limit or avoid conflicts of interest.[38–40] Other policies are needed to monitor and deal promptly with scientific fraud and to rehabilitate, whenever possible, scientists who violate the common understanding of what is acceptable behavior. A morally responsive scientific community will insist on close supervision of assistants and students, will provide protection for "whistle blowers," and will link authorship and accountability for research publications.

The National Academy of Sciences has been concerned that science retain its privilege of self-governance. An Academy panel has suggested that one way to do this is to establish a separate body, outside of academia, to set ethical standards. Dr. David, chairman of the panel, is quoted as saying, "We must assure the people who pay for the work, such as the Congress, that there is some reason to believe that we are doing things right and that we are not cheating." An ethically responsive community would do well to follow David's advice.[41]

By these measures, the character of the whole body of scientists can be gradually improved and its moral sensitivities heightened. We then might talk even of the virtuous institution of science. Then, when the moral and intellectual values of scholarly research come into conflict with the values of the industrial model, fewer compromises will be made in the name of exigency.[42]

There are practical implications in the establishment of a sense of moral community among scientists with a common understanding of the virtues requisite for achieving the goods internal to the practice of research. Every policy and action of science and scientists would have to meet a more stringent ethical test.

For example, most conflict-of-interest policies forbid faculty members to own equity in a company that might benefit from their research. One medical school, however, has gone the other way. It joins its faculty entrepreneurs by becoming partners in the commercialization of research results. This policy, it is asserted, reduces faculty–university conflict (indeed) and protects the public. Would such a policy pass muster with a body of scientists who had developed an ethic of moral sensitivity?[43] Could such an ethic countenance the stonewalling and persistent denial of wrong-doing and responsibility by senior scientists for fraud in their laboratories?[44] Or the relative silence of their colleagues? Or the outcry from the biomedical research community at the announcement of new conflict-of-interest rules by the NIH, or closing the Office of Scientific Integrity?[45]

Clearly, there is a collective responsibility and accountability on the part of the entire scientific community. When serious misconduct occurs, it reflects a breakdown in the moral values of that community that should be supportive of scientific integrity and censorious of moral lapses that damage the whole purpose of research. Education in ethics will not be a radical cure, but it is a step in the direction of the kind of moral accountability that Congress and the public require if we are to avoid the kind of control that will frustrate the very purposes of scientific research, to the ultimate detriment of our whole society.

Conclusion

Recurrent disclosures of scientific fraud, conflict-of-interest, and other forms of misconduct have cast a shadow over the moral integrity of the research enterprise. Congress and the public are asking seriously if science can be left to govern itself. There are forebodings in current congressional investigations of serious legal and regulatory constraints on the conduct of research. The integrity of science and the benefits of research to society are seriously threatened.

If research is to be safeguarded against these eventualities, the onus of responsibility rests with the scientific community. It must give evidence of its moral probity. Rather than denying or trivializing misconduct, we must accept moral accountability for it. Rather than demanding freedom, we must earn it. We must confront the ineluctable fact that the scientific community holds its freedom and support in trust. Similarly, the doctor–patient relationship relies on integrity and trust. If the freedom to be creative about clinical healing as well as scientific research is abused, all physicians and scientists are morally diminished and society may justly intervene.

Even in today's complicated milieu of industrialization, commercialization, and corporatization of research, the final determinant of the quality of research remains the character and conscience of the scientists. We must return to the ethics of personal responsibility, the most ancient branch of ethics, the ethics of character and virtue. Paradoxically, by taking the moral high road even at the risk of non-survival, we take the surest road to survival.

Notes

1. P. Alan Dioisopoulos, and Craig R. Ducat, *The Right to Privacy: Essays and Cases* (St. Paul, MN: West Publishing Co., 1976).

2. Pierce v. Society of Sisters. 268 U.S. 510 (1925); Loving v. Virginia, 388 U.S. 1 (1967); West Virginia State Board v. Barnette, 319 U.S. 624 (1943); Eisenstadt v. Baird, 405 U.S. 438 (1972); Roe v. Wade, 410 U.S. 113 (1973); Griswold v. Connecticut, 381 U.S. 479 (1965).

3. Schoendorff v. Society of New York Hospitals, 211 N.Y. 125, 126, 105 N.E. 92, 93 (1914).

4. *In re* Quinlan, 70 N.J. 10, 355 A. 2d 647 (1976); In re Eichner, 52 N. Y. 2d 363, 420 N.E.2d 64, 428 N.Y.S.2d 266, cert. denied, 454 U.S. 858 (1981); In re Conroy, 98 N.J. 321, 486 A.2d 1209 (1985); Bouvia v. Superior Court (Glenchur), 179 Cal. App. 3d 1127, 225 Cal. Rptr. 297 (Ct. App. 1886) review denied (Cal. June 5, 1986); In re Jobes, 108 N.J. 394, 529 A.2d 434 (1987); Brophy v. New England Sinai Hospital, Inc., 398 Mass. 417, 497 N.E.2d 626 (1986).

5. John Locke, *A Second Treatise of Government,* 3d ed. (Oxford: Blackwell, 1966).

6. Immanuel Kant, *Groundwork for the Metaphysics of Morals,* trans. and analyzed by H.J. Paton (New York: Harper and Row, 1964).

7. Ibid., p. 103.

8. Ibid., p. 105.

9. Ibid., p. 107.

10. President's Commission for the Study of Ethical Problems in Medicine and Biomedical and Behavioral Research, *Report of the President's Commission for the Study of Ethical Problems in Medical and Biomedical and Behavioral Research: Deciding to Forego Life-Sustaining Treatment* (Washington, DC: General Printing Office, 1983).

11. For example, in the Illinois Surrogate Decision Act of 1991.

12. Ruth R. Faden and Tom L. Beauchamp, *A History and Theory of Informed Consent* (New York: Oxford University Press, 1986).

13. Edmund D. Pellegrino, and David C. Thomasma, *For the Patient's Good: The Restoration of Beneficence in Health Care* (New York: Oxford University Press, 1988).

14. Thomas Jefferson to Peter Carr, August 19, 1785, in *The Papers of Thomas Jefferson,* Vol. 8, ed. Julian P. Boyd (Princeton, NJ: Princeton University Press, 1953), pp. 406.

15. Henry K. Beecher, "Ethics and Clinical Research," *New England Journal of Medicine* 274 (1966):1354–1360.

16. Philip Handler, *Fraud in Biomedical Research: Hearings Before the Subcommittee on Investigation and Oversight of the Committee on Science and Technology, U.S. House of Representatives* (Washington, DC: U.S. Government Printing Office, 1981), p. 12.

17. Gerald Dworkin, "Fraud and Science," *Research Ethics,* ed. Kare Berg, Knut Erik Tranoy, and A. R. Liss (New York: Alan R. Liss, Inc., 1983), pp. 65–74.

18. Paul Feyerabend, *Against Method* (London: Verso, 1975).

19. William Broad and Nicholas Wade, *Betrayers of the Trust* (New York: Simon & Schuster, 1982).

20. Ibid.

21. Handler, *Fraud,* p. 12.

22. Lewis Thomas, "Falsity and Failure," *Discover* (June 1981):38–39.

23. The Nuremburg Code (1947), reprinted in *Biomedical Ethics,* ed. T. A. Mapps and J. S. Zembaty (New York: McGraw-Hill, 1981), p. 145.

24. The Declaration of Helsinki (1964), revised in 1975, in Mappes and Zembaty, *Biomedical Ethics,* pp. 146–147.

25. *Proposed International Guidelines for Research Involving Human Subjects* (Geneva and Albany, N.Y.: World Health Organization and the Council for International Organizations of Medical Sciences, 1982).

26. Tom L. Beauchamp and James F. Childress, *Principles of Biomedical Ethics,* 3d ed. (New York: Oxford University Press, 1989).

27. Alasdair MacIntyre, "The Return to Virtue Ethics," *The Twenty-Fifth Anniversary of Vatican II, A Look Back and a Look Ahead,* ed. Russell E. Smith (Braintree, MA: The Pope John Center, 1990), pp. 239–249.

28. Alasdair MacIntyre, *After Virtue,* 2d ed. (Notre Dame, IN: University of Notre Dame Press, 1984).

29. Ibid., pp. 174–179.

30. Ibid., pp. 206–207.

31. Aristotle, *Nicomachean Ethics,* 1168a28–34 and ll68bl–38.

32. A very recent example is HR-1819.102, U.S. Congress, April 16, 1991, which seeks to prevent financial conflicts of interest and make data available to other researchers.

33. Edmund D. Pellegrino, "Beneficence, Scientific Autonomy and Self-Interest: Ethical Dilemmas in Clinical Research," *Georgetown Medicine* 1(1) (Spring 1991):21–28.

34. H. K. Beecher, *Experimentation in Man* (Springfield, IL: Thomas, 1959).

35. Ruth Faden and Tom Beauchamp, *Informed Consent* (New York: Oxford University Press, 1986).

36. Edmund D. Pellegrino, "Teaching Medical Ethics: Some Persistent Questions and Some Responses," *Academic Medicine, The Journal of the Association of American Medical Colleges* 64(12)(December 1989):701–703.

37. Edmund D. Pellegrino and Thomas K. McElhinney, *Teaching Ethics, The Humanities, and Human Values in Medical Schools: A Ten-Year Overview* (Washington, DC: Institute on Human Values in Medicine, Society for Health and Human Values, 1982).

38. *The Maintenance of Ethical Standards in the Conduct of Research* (Washington, D.C.: Association of American Medical Colleges, June 24, 1982).

39. *Conflicts of Interest in Academic Health Centers* (Washington, DC: Association of Academic Health Centers, 1990).

40. Eliot Marshall, "Harvard's Tough New Rules," *Science* 248 (April 13, 1990):154.

41. Philip J. Hilts, "Panel Urges Independent Body to Set Ethical Standards in Service," *New York Times* (March 28, 1991):4.

42. Eliot Marshall, "When Commerce and Academe Collide," *Science* 248 (April 13, 1990):152–156.

43. William B. Neaves and Kern Wildenthal, *Conflict of Interest Issues Surrounding Faculty Participation in the Ownership of Technology and Drug Companies* (abstract) (Washington, DC: Fidia Research Foundation Conference, April 29–30, 1991), p. 22.

44. Theresa Imanishi-Kari and David Baltimore, "Stonewalling," *Science* 251 (1991):1552–1553. See also David Hamilton, "Baltimore Throws in the Towel," *Science* 252 (1991):768–770.

45. G. Christopher Anderson, "Research Ethics: No Conflicts-of-Interests Rules," *Nature* 343 (January 11, 1990):104.

12

Self-Effacement

One of the least popular virtues of our time in medicine must be the virtue of self-effacement. Because of the tremendous narcissism of our age and the power of medicine we discussed in Chapter 10, putting others and their needs first is a difficult task. The professions today are afflicted with a species of moral malaise that may prove fatal to their moral identities and perilous to our whole society. The malaise is manifest in a growing conviction, even among conscientious doctors, that it is no longer possible to practice their professions within traditional ethical constraints. For reasons that are explained below, this discussion focuses on medicine and obliquely considers the other learned professions, law and ministry. More specifically, the belief is taking hold that unless they look out for their own interests, professionals will be crushed by the forces of commercialization, competition, government regulation, malpractice, advertising, public and media hostility, and a host of other inimical socio-economic forces.

These forces, it is asserted, are conspiring to transform the learned professions into crafts, businesses, or technologies. They are beyond the control of the professions. The fault lies not with the professions. Unless there is some upheaval in conventional morality, professional ethics as we have known it has no future. Indeed, perhaps given the realities of professional practice, professional ethics has rested on faulty philosophical foundations from its very beginnings. This line of reasoning leads to the conclusion that the self-interest of the professional justifies the compromises in, and even the rejection of, obligations imposed by traditional concepts of professional ethics.

In this chapter, strong exception is taken to this line of reasoning both in its foundations and in its conclusions. We argue to the contrary: (1) that what deficiencies exist in professional morality are, as they have always been, deficiencies in character and virtue; (2) that a firm philosophical foundation exists for altruism and **fidelity to trust** in the ethics of the professions; (3) that professional ethics must at times be independent of conventional morality; and (4) that the professions are moral communities with enormous moral power that, properly used, can sustain the moral integrity of the practitioner and professions. Moreover, if they use their moral power well, the professions can become paradigms of disinterested service that can raise the level of conventional morality.

This is an ambitious set of assertions. To speak of character and virtue in today's moral climate is to be suspected of sanctimoniousness or hypocrisy. We must admit that the concepts of virtue and character are two of the oldest and most slippery in moral philosophy. Also, the proper place of self-interest in virtue ethics has never been satisfactorily settled. Finally, we still lack a coherent moral philosophy of the professions in which to locate the concepts of character, altruism, and self-interest and to define the relationships between them. These difficulties notwithstanding, we cannot avoid engagement with what we take to be the central crisis in medicine today—the confusion about who and what physicians are, and what they should be.

The Moral Malaise of the Professions

The moral malaise to which we refer centers on more subtle issues than those more egregious infractions of professional ethics that everyone will condemn. There is no need, therefore, to list a jeremiad of gross immorality like incompetence, fraud, deception, mismanagement of funds, violations of confidentiality, or sexual abuse of clients or patients. The more immediate concern is with those practices that are more at the "moral margin."[1] These practices are often legal, often socially acceptable, and often tolerated, though with some misgivings. They occupy a moral gray zone where the interests of the professional and the patient or client intersect and where the vulnerability of the latter makes him exploitable by the former. They are ethical "ozone holes" that open up when moral sensitivities are blunted. Like their physical counterparts at the Earth's poles, ethical ozone holes can spread and have dire consequences unless repaired.

Each profession has its own list of morally questionable practices that its members would justify on the grounds of threatened self-interest. We will list a few from the medical profession and leave to the readers in others to fill in their own analogues. For medicine, we would select these examples: refusing to treat patients with HIV infection for fear of contagion; denying service to the poor and those with inadequate or exhausted insurance benefits; turning away complicated cases from the emergency room for fear of malpractice suits; cooperating with hospital or public policies that require early discharge; economic transfer or the "dumping" of those who cannot pay on other hospitals; the various forms of medical entrepreneurism like investment in health care facilities; for-profit medical ventures of all sorts; marketing to increase the demand for dubious or unnecessary treatment or tests; accepting bonuses for denying needed care; and enjoying the many emoluments proffered by pharmaceutical companies.

Other professions can draw up their own lists of morally dubious practices. All such practices, however, have three features in common. First, they are based on the use of privilege and power for the personal gain of the professional. Second, they reflect a failure to take certain risks required for the well-being of those whom the profession serves. Finally, in the case of both of these features, justification is sought on the grounds of legitimate self-interest. These practices and the justification sought for them derive from the deemphasis on character and virtue in the medical professions.

In what follows, we will examine three questions about the current moral malaise of the professions: (1) What are the reasons for the erosion of virtue ethics and the moral legitimation of self-interest in the ethics of the professions? (2) Is there a philosophical basis for restoring virtue ethics of the professions? (3) What are the practical and theoretical implications of such a return of virtue ethics? Before examining these questions, We should define the sense in which we shall use each of the key terms in this chapter.

Definitions of Key Terms

Virtue

We have examined the definition of virtue in general and of specific virtues in particular throughout this book. Here we offer a summary of the definition of virtue. Virtue makes us function well as humans to achieve our purposes. We are thereby made good humans. Defining human excellence is more difficult than defining the excellence of a knife. Aristotle addresses that question in both *Nicomachean Ethics* and *Eudemian Ethics*. What is important in that discussion is that Aristotle's definition of virtue is linked to two other concepts—the concepts of the nature and the good of man. It is the fragmentation of the unity among these concepts that is largely responsible for the confusion we experience today in arriving at some consensus about the meaning of virtue. Plato, Aristotle, and the Stoics were in general agreement, as was Aquinas (with the additional consideration of humanity's spiritual nature), on a comprehensive moral philosophy of which virtue was a part. The postmedieval dissolution of this moral philosophy, which we shall shortly examine, has left the idea of virtue without roots.

It is very difficult to attempt to define the virtuous person, the one who possesses to a high degree the character traits that make for a good person. We do believe it is possible to define the virtues that make for a good physician, lawyer, or clergyperson in terms of the ends to which those professions are dedicated.

Character

The term "character" may be taken in two ways. In a general sense, it summates the kind of person one is, as revealed by the virtues and vices one exhibits in one's attitudes and actions. More specifically, a person of character is one who can predictably be trusted to act well in most circumstances, to consider others in her decisions, to look at the long-term meanings of immediate impulses, and to order those impulses according to the canons of morality. In Aristotle's sense, a person of character (and here we mean virtuous character) is one who "stands well" with reference to the passions, who does not yield to extremes of self-interest, pleasure, or the desire for power.

Ethics of the Professions

By "ethics of the professions," we do not mean the norms actually followed by professionals or the professional codes they espouse, but rather the moral obligations deductible from the kinds of activity in which they are engaged. The ethics of the professions, therefore, consists in a rational and systematic ordering of the principles, rules, duties, and virtues intrinsic to achieving the ends to which a profession is dedicated. This is the "internal morality" of a profession.[2]

Profession

By a "profession," we mean something more than the usual sociological definition. A profession is, literally speaking, a declaration of a way of life that is specific, a way of life in which expert knowledge is used not primarily for personal gain but for the benefit of those who need that knowledge. The fuller meaning of this definition will emerge as our line of argument unfolds.

Altruism and Self-Interest

"Altruism" and "self-interest," as we shall use these terms in this chapter, are opposing moral concepts. Without entering into a detailed history of these two ideas, we would make the following distinctions. Altruism is the trait that disposes a person to take the interests of others into account in using power, privilege, position, and knowledge. It was first introduced by August Comte (1798–1857). One need not accept Comte's philosophy of humanity and his positivism to use the term as we do. The key term for the ethics of the professions is "altruistic beneficence." This means not only taking the interests of others into account but doing so in such a fashion that our intentions and acts give some degree of preference to the intention of others. This is a more elevated notion of beneficence than simple benevolence, or wishing others well, and nonmaleficence, or not doing them harm. It implies some degree of effacement of self-interest. Altruistic beneficence is particularly important for the professions given the special phenomenology of the professional relationship, which we define later.

Self-interest, too, has several meanings. There is a legitimate self-interest that pertains to the duties we owe to ourselves—duties that guard health, life, some measure of material well-being, the good of our families, friends, and so on. Aristotle made clear the two senses in which self-love may exist in humans.[3] There is also an illegitimate sense of self-interest—at least in the moral philosophy of virtue—and that is selfish self-interest. This may be legitimate when taking into account that the good of others involves heroic degrees of self-sacrifice to the point of discomfort, financial loss, harm to one's family, or even death. Whether degrees of altruistic beneficence that require some cost in time, effort, or discomfort are required in ordinary affairs is a debatable question.

The major point in the argument, however, is that, given the nature of professional relationships, some effacement of self-interest—which we shall take to mean the same as beneficent altruism—is morally obligatory for health professionals. A virtuous professional, then, is one who can be expected with reasonable certainty to exhibit as one trait of character altruistic beneficence construed as effacement of self-interest. The precise limits of such a trait, the way in which it would be defined in a specific instance, is not definable by formula.

While we focus here on medicine, and relatedly on law and the ministry, other occupations like teaching and the military have been called professions in the past, and now almost every activity that requires skill and is done for a living is called a profession. Indeed, some of the features described for the learned three are possessed by other occupations. But the traditional three are paradigms of professional ethics because the characteristics that define them are clustered in a unique way as to degree, kind, and number. To the extent that other professions commit themselves to other than self-interest, they approach the paradigm professions, and what we say applies analogically to them.

The Erosion of Virtue and the Rise of Self-Interest

What accounts for the erosion of virtue ethics? There are at least four factors in the answer to this question: (1) the unresolved conceptual tension between virtue and self-interest; (2) the conceptual difficulties of virtue ethics itself; (3) the modern turn in ethics from the character of the moral agent to the resolution of dilemmas; and (4) the shift in economic and political values in the last decade.

The Inherent Tension Between Virtue and Self-Interest

The tension between self-interest and virtue was recognized at the beginning of Western moral philosophy. Plato has Socrates confront this dilemma in *The Republic* when Thrasymachus asserts that "justice is simply the interest of the stronger."[4] Glaucon, for his part, contends that man by nature pursues self-interest and is deflected only by law—an idea also advanced by other ethical "relativists" like Thucydides and Gorgias. Callicles goes further and insists that virtue consists in acting selfishly and tyrannically. William K. C. Guthrie shows how persistent the idea of self-interest and self-love was in the thought of the Sophists.[5] Aristotle too has difficulties with the reality of self-interest and its reconciliation with his doctrine of moral virtue. He asks if one should love oneself primarily or one's neighbor.[6] At one point, he tries to show, like so many philosophers thereafter, that acting to benefit others contributes to happiness and therefore is in one's own self-interest.[7] But this is a weak argument because Aristotle also asserts that the truly virtuous person ought to practice altruism for its own sake.[8] In his interesting analysis of this problem in Books VIII and IX of the *Eudeman Ethics,* Engberg-Pedersen concludes that Aristotle's position is that justice is the basis of all the virtues. The virtuous person assigns no more of natural goods to himself than to others. In this way he encompasses altruism, places restraints on inordinate self-interest, and serves legitimate self-interest.[9]

Despite the unresolved difficulties of dealing with the reality of self-interest, the ethics of Aristotle, Plato, and the Stoics placed the emphasis squarely on virtues. Virtue ethics dominated classical and Hellenistic moral philosophy. It came to its highest development in the moral philosophy of Aquinas, who joined the supernatural to the natural virtues. Thus the classical and medieval philosophies of virtue constituted a continuum.

This continuum centered on the conception of the virtuous person as one who exhibited the traits of character essential to human flourishing, and to optimal fulfillment of the capabilities inherent in human nature. For such a person, self-interest was recognized as a responsibility, but it was to be submerged to varying degrees of noble acts in the interests of others. The good life called for a rational balance between personal good and the good of others.[10] But the cardinal virtues—temperance, justice, courage, and prudence—all implied some degree of effacement of self-interest as a mark of the virtuous person. At a minimum, the virtuous person was not to take advantage of the vulnerability of others. As examples: Socrates chose death to teach a moral lesson to his fellow Athenians; Plato distinguished the art of making money from the art of healing;[11] and Cicero admonished the corn merchant not to raise prices when the crop wa small.[12] Hippocrates makes beneficent concern for the welfare of patients the first principle of medical ethics.[13] Thus, while they recognized the reality of self-interest, the ancient and medieval moral philosophers held firmly to virtue as the touchstone of the moral life.

In the postmedieval period, two philosophical assaults were launched on virtue ethics, one by Machiavelli and the other by Thomas Hobbes. Both are conceptual descendants of Thrasymachus, Callicles, and the antivirtue pre-Socratics. Both replaced the optimistic view of human nature with moral pessimism. Both found the traditional concepts of virtue antithetical to human nature and self-interest. Machiavelli simply converted the traditional virtues into vices, while Hobbes psychologized them as a form of self-interest. The Machiavellian and Hobbesian strains are the heart of today's moral malaise and cynicism, which seek to give moral legitimacy to the professional's self-interest.

The Machiavellian Strain

Machiavelli (1469–1527) was too well educated in classical humanism to deny totally the virtue as an ideal in human conduct. But the observation of the real world in which men lived—in warfare, tyranny, and political upheaval—convinced him that there was no survival value in living virtuously. The good man simply could not thrive in a world in which so many others were not good.[14] And so Machiavelli advised the prince who would be successful to use whatever means would ensure his survival and the continuance of his power. The classical cardinal virtues of temperance, justice—even, at times, fortitude and prudence—could be impediments when dealing with those who ignored these constraints on self-interest. In these circumstances, the virtues thus became vices. Moreover, in the Machiavellian view, virtue itself became an instrumental notion, a power to effect a given end rather than a behavioral ideal. Indeed, for Machiavelli, virtue became *viri,* "manliness"—an expression of power, rather than a disposition to act well, as it was understood in the classical-medieval continuum.

Bernard Mandeville (1670–1773), a physician, went further than Machiavelli in some ways. Not only did he think the virtues were impractical, but he held them to be vices—destructive not only for personal but also for social good. It is through greed, the desire for luxury, pleasure, and power, that society prospers and things get done. The satisfaction of acquisitiveness, intemperance, and gluttony creates jobs, puts money into the economy, and provides a livelihood for many.[15] Mandeville's *Fable of the Bees,* whether tongue-in-cheek or not, has been influential in encouraging an antivirtue bias that has always found supporters and has many today.

Nietzsche's (1844–1900) antivirtue stance was of a different kind, but still in the Machiavellian spirit. For Nietzsche's *Uebermensch,* the traditional virtues were meaningless. They were simply impediments to the achievement of greatness. The virtues were for lesser mortals. For the superman, virtues like temperance or justice would be vices.[16]

A more modern exponent of a similar moral viewpoint is Ayn Rand. Her ideas, though far less well-argued than those of Machiavelli, Mandeville, or Nietzsche, are a current compound of all three. Rand's novels of the successful architect or industrialist extol the "virtues" of individualism, ruthlessness, power, and uninhibited pursuit of wealth and self-interest.[17] Her ideas have had a considerable influence on those who seek moral justification for their acquisitive instincts. In this regard, it is interesting to note that the slogan of *Regardie's* magazine is "Money, Power, Greed."

Moral Machiavellianism—whether in its original version or in its later varieties in Mandeville, Nietzsche, or Rand—is very much alive today. We see it in the medical entrepreneurs who own hospital or nursing homes, in the lawyer/power broker who sells influence or leveraged buyouts; and in the multi-million-dollar electronic ministries. Indeed, all who hold that virtue simply does not pay and that it is a fool's enterprise are moral Machiavellians.

The Hobbesian Strain

Machiavelli made the virtues into vices. Thomas Hobbes (1588–1679), on the other hand, tried to maintain some idea of virtue that was recognizable and yet to reconcile it with self-interest. His was a formal philosophical break with the medieval tradition. His aim was to establish ethics on purely naturalistic grounds, free of the theological spirit that characterized the medieval synthesis. He built his moral philosophy on a pessimistic view of human nature that departed sharply from the essentially optimistic classical-medieval view.

Aristotle opens his *Politics* by asserting that man is a social animal. Man, Hobbes said, is unsocial by nature. He enters society only to satisfy his most fundamental urges. His selfishness is primary and is expressed in a desire to preserve his own life, enhance pleasure, avoid pain, and become secure from attack by others. Hobbes does not make the virtues into vices; rather, he puts them at the service of self-interest. We pity others because we see the possibility of being in the position of those we pity. We are benevolent in return. "All society," he said, "is for gain or glory."[18] We obey society's rules only because we feel that if we do not, others will threaten our security. In Hobbes' view, effacement of self-interest is unnatural, because it makes us the victims of others. Self-interest determines what is good and bad. But self-interest alone will not secure a peaceable society. That must finally be secured by an absolute sovereign, or society will be torn apart by competing self-interests.

Hobbes' view of self-interest was coupled with a scorn for the idea of the good, which had been vital to classical and medieval philosophy. If the good is reducible to what we like or dislike, as Hobbes suggested, then virtues and vices are also matters of preference. Hobbes' powerful assertions shaped much of English moral philosophy. His successors tried either to rebut the primacy of self-interest or to reconcile it with some more altruistic principle. John Locke (1632–1704), for example, agreed with Hobbes that good and evil are determined by pain or pleasure or conformity to some law. He did assert that we ought to help others, but only if it did not endanger our own self-interest. Shaftesbury (1671–1713) tried hard to show that self-interest and service to others were synonymous. Virtues, he said, pay off in self-interest because of the pleasure we get from benevolent acts. The vices like anger, intemperance, and covetousness, on the other hand, bring pain. Shaftesbury thought that we ought to embrace virtue because we have an obligation to protect self-interest, so that affection for virtue is really affection for self-interest. Hutcheson (1694–1746) developed Shaftesbury's moral sense (theory) more fully, as did Hume (1711–1776). They identified virtue as that which gives the spectator of virtuous acts a feeling of approbation, while vicious acts elicit disapproval. They took some of the bluntness out of Hobbes' emphasis on self-interest. But they ended up agreeing that we have no ultimate obligation to virtue other than its bearing on our self-interest or happiness. Adam Smith (1723–1790) held that virtues are those traits of character that are useful or agreeable to the moral sentiment of the agent or others. Bentham (1748–1832) argued that whatever is conducive to the general happiness always conduces to the happiness of the agent. In this way, his utilitarianism reconciles self-regarding and other-regarding interests by subsuming all of these interests under the principle of greatest happiness. J. S. Mill (1806–1873) went further than Bentham, positing that the greatest good of all is the source of one's own happiness. One's own self-interest, therefore, is best served by acting for the good of all. According to this view, consciously doing without happiness to achieve the greatest good of all is paradoxically, a source of happiness.[19]

In contrast to the moral sentiment theorists, and the utilitarians, the Cambridge intuitionists like Cudworth (1617–1688) Henry More (1614–1687), and Cumberland (1631–1718) tried to show that there were reasons for virtuous acts even if they conflicted with self-interest. More even postulated a ''Boniform faculty,'' a virtue that gives us mastery over our basic impulses to serve selfish interests first.[20]

Bishop Joseph Butler (1692–1752) took issue with both Shaftesbury and Hobbes. Neither self-love not benevolence was the only affection involved in human behavior. Altruism and self-interest do not completely exclude other desires and motivations. Nor are benevolence and self-interest mutually exclusive. Man has a conscience that enables him to order his passions so that he can do what is good not just for the self. By conscience man can know how much benevolence will advance and how much it will damage his self-interest. Butler was a cleric and looked to God to implant conscience in humans to point out what action is most in conformity with human nature. Thus conscience enables us to know that some things are inherently good and others inherently bad. Butler thus invoked theology implicitly, if not always explicitly, though he tried, as did Hobbes, to extract his moral philosophy from reason.[21]

Enough has been said to demonstrate how the question of altruism and self-interest arose in Hobbes and Machiavelli and established two powerful strains of thought with which moral philosophy has been occupied ever since. As pointed out earlier, the problem arose in ancient philosophy as well. In Christian moral philosophy as enunciated by Aquinas, self-preservation was built into natural law. What is owed to oneself and what is owed to others is ordered by the virtue of charity, which entails love for others as children of God and not for any ulterior purpose. This is the message of the Sermon on the Mount. Indeed, it may be that this is the only way in which the inherent tensions between self-interest and altruism can ever be finally resolved.

These tensions certainly have not been resolved in twentieth-century moral philosophy. The subjectivism and emotivism of Ayer, the prescriptivism of Hare, and the existentialism of Sartre all make moral judgment matters of approval or disapproval, preference or self-determination. The metaethical emphasis on the language and logic of moral discourse, rather than on the content of moral judgments, further weakened the classical notions of virtues. As a result, the definition of virtue has become either so vague as to be meaningless or so encompassing as to include every conceivable likable trait.[22]

Twentieth-century moralists have refined the eighteenth-century notion of moral sentiment and further psychologized ethics. In light of the psychology of Freud and the behaviorism of Watson or Skinner today, many moralists look to modern psychology to define the virtues and to close the gap between knowing the good and being motivated to do the good. Others look to genetics, culture, or social organization to explain altruism and self-interest.[23] Nagel, on the other hand, presents a challenge to this trend and argues for the rationality of altruism. In doing so, he rejects the human subordination of reason to desire or emotion.[24] Philippa Foot tries unsuccessfully to link virtue and self-interest in her work on virtues and vices.[25]

The disarray of normative ethics, including the destruction of virtue ethics, has occasioned a spate of recent attempts to resuscitate the classical and especially the Aristotelian idea of virtue. This move was initiated by Anscombe[26] and MacIntyre,[27] and their success varies. The extent to which they can reverse the dominance of self-interest in ethics begun by Hobbes is highly problematic.

Conceptual Difficulties of a Virtue-Based Ethics

The second major factor in the erosion of virtue ethics is the philosophical difficulty inherent in the concept of virtue itself. The first problem is its lack of specificity. Virtue ethics does not tell us how to resolve specific moral dilemmas. It deemphasizes principles, rules, duties, and concrete prescriptions. It only says that the virtuous person will be disposed to act in accord with the virtue appropriate to the situation. This lack of specificity leads to a distressing circularity in reasoning. The right and the good is that which the virtuous person would do, and the virtuous person is one who would do the right and the good. We must define either the right and the good or the virtuous person if we are to break out of this logical impasse. But these are just the definitions that have defied the conceptual ingenuity of the world's best philosophers. Furthermore, virtue theory cannot stand apart from some theory of human nature and the good. The more vague our definitions of human nature and its *telos,* the more difficult it is to keep virtue from becoming vice and vice virtue. Since virtue ethics puts its emphasis on the character of the agent, it requires a consistent philosophical anthropology; otherwise, it easily becomes subjectivist, emotivist, relativist, and self-destructive.

Further difficulties include the relations of intent to outward behavior. Is good intention a criterion of a virtuous person? How do we determine intention? Can a good intention absolve the agent of responsibility for an act that ends in harm—for example, a physician telling a patient the truth out of the virtue of honesty, precipitating a serious depression or even suicide? Few persons are virtuous all the time. How many lapses move us from the virtuous to the vision category? How does virtue ethics connect with duty and principle-based ethics, which give the objectivity virtue seems to lack?

Classical ethics in the East and the West have usually eschewed systems of rules or principles, or at least have subordinated them to the notion of moral character. Where do virtue and supererogation meet? Are virtues synonymous with duties? Is supererogation merely a higher degree of virtue? Why are some people virtuous and other not? Must we turn to sociobiology for the answer, as some suggest?[28] Are virtues genetically ingrained, mere survival mechanisms designed to propagate the gene pool?

In spite of their ancient lineage, these fundamental questions are yet to be answered. Because they have not been answered to everyone's satisfaction, moralists have turned to something more probable—to the questions What shall I do? How do I solve the dilemma before me now?

The Turn to Quandary Solving

This brings us to the third point regarding the erosion of virtue ethics, namely, the turn—particularly in professional ethics—toward quandary and dilemma solving. This is the result of a number of factors operating in the last two decades. One is the concreteness and urgency of the new ethical issues arising from scientific advance and sociopolitical change. Medical and biological progress, for example, challenges traditional ethics; yet, they must be confronted without the ethical compass points of a consensus on values or common religious beliefs. We are now a morally heterogeneous society, divided on the most fundamental ethical issues, particularly about the meaning of life and death. Without a common conception of human nature, we cannot agree on what constitutes a good life and the virtues that ought to characterize it. As a result, the ethics of the professions, especially of the medical profession, have turned to the analysis of dilemmas and of the process of ethical decision making. For many, ethics consists primarily of balancing rights, duties, and prima facie principles and the resolution of conflicts among them. Procedural ethics has replaced normative ethics. This avoids the impasses generated when patients, clients, and professionals hold fundamentally opposing moral viewpoints.

Yet analysis cannot substitute for character and virtue, even though it provides conceptual clarity. Moral acts are the acts of human agents. Their quality is determined by the characters of the persons doing the analysis. Character shapes the way we define a moral problem, selects what we think is an ethical issue, and decides which principles, values, and technical details are determinative.

It makes a great difference, therefore, whether a professional is motivated by self-interest or altruism. Given the realities of professional relationships, the character of the professional cannot be eliminated from its central position. That is why virtue ethics must be restored as the keystone of the ethics of the professions.

A fourth and final factor eroding a virtue approach in the medical profession is the legitimation in public attitudes of and tolerance for self-interest in response to the economic imperatives acting so forcefully on the health care system. To this end, physicians and other providers have been encouraged to compete with each other. The availability, cost, and quality of health services have been turned over increasingly to market forces. The Federal Trade Commission has classified the professions as businesses and made them subject to one ordering principle—the preservation of competition.[29] Health providers have been encouraged to become entrepreneurs, to invest in health care facilities and technologies, to be offered bonuses for keeping utilization of health care resources to a minimum. Without these incentives, it is argued, the best persons will not enter medicine or will retire early. Medical progress would stop and new services would cease to be available. For the first time in medical history, self-interest has been given legal and moral legitimation and profit has been turned into a professional virtue. These trends are making the physician into a businessperson, and entrepreneur, a proletarian, a gatekeeper, and a bureaucrat. Never has there been more confusion about who and what it is to be a physician.

The Philosophical Basis for Restoring a Virtue Ethics

Is there a sound philosophical foundation in the nature of professional activity for resolving the tension between altruism and self-interest in favor of virtue and character? We think there is. We ground a proposal in six characteristics of the relationship of professionals with those who seek their help. Individually, none of these phenomena is unique in kind or degree. They may exist individually in other human relationships and occupations.

But as a moral cluster they are, in fact, unique and generate a kind of internal morality, a grounding for the ethics of the professions that is in some way impervious to vacillations in philosophical fashions, as well as social, economic, or political change. This internal morality explains why the ethics of medicine, for example, remained until two decades ago firmly rooted in the ethics of character and virtue. This was true of the medical ethics of the Hippocratic school and the Stoics, and it is found in the seminal texts of Moslem, Jewish, and Christian medical moralists. It persisted in the eighteenth century in the writing of John Gregory, Thomas Percival, and Samuel Bard, who, although cognizant of the philosophies of Hobbes, Adam Smith, and Hume, nonetheless maintained the traditional dedication of the profession to the welfare of the patient and to a certain set of virtues. Only in the last two decades has there been (to use Hume's terms) a "sentiment of approbation" regarding self-interest.

The first distinguishing characteristic of professional relationships is the dependence, **vulnerability**, and eminent exploitability of the person who seeks the help of a physician, lawyer, or clergy. The person in need of help to restore health, receive justice, or rectify his relationship with God is anxious, in distress, and driven by fear. To avoid death, damnation, or incarceration, he is impelled to seek help, though he wishes he could avoid it. He is not free to pursue life's other goals until help is forthcoming.

The second characteristic of professional relationships is their **inherent inequality**. The professional possesses the knowledge that the patient or client needs. This places the preponderance of power in her hands. She can use it well or poorly, for good or evil, for service or self-interest. How can we speak, as some do, of the professional relationship as a contract when one party is so dependent upon the other's services?

The third characteristic of professional relationships is their special **fiduciary character**. In a state of vulnerability[30] and inequality, we are forced to trust our physicians, lawyers, or pastors. We are ill equipped to evaluate their competence. We are forced to reveal our intimate selves—baring our bodies, our personal lives, our souls, and our failings to another person who is a stranger. Without these invasions of our privacy, we cannot be healed or helped. Moreover, the professional invites our trust. Professionals begin their relationship with us with the question "How can I help you?" Implicitly they are saying "I have the knowledge you need; trust me to have it and to use it in your best interests." In the case of medicine, that promise is made in a public oath at the time of graduation when the graduate announces to all present that, henceforth, he can be trusted to serve interests other than his own. It is repeated in the codes of medicine and the other professions and in the ordination rites of clergymen.

Indeed, it is the public declaration that defines a true profession and separates it from other occupations. The very word "profession" comes from the Latin *profiteri,* to declare aloud, to accept publicly a special way of life, one that promises that the profession can be trusted to act in other than its own interest. Business people and crafts people ask to be trusted, but not at a cost to themselves. *Caveat emptor* can never be the first principle of a profession.

Fourth, **the knowledge** of true professionals cannot be wholly proprietary. Their knowledge is ordained to a practical end, to meeting certain fundamental human needs. Professional knowledge does not exist for its own sake. This is clearest in medicine, where society permits invasions of privacy that would otherwise be criminal in order that physicians may be trained. Thus, medical students who are not fully skilled are permitted to dissect human bodies, attend and assist at autopsies and operations, and participate in the care of sick people. They are allowed literally to practice, albeit under supervision. Surgeons in training take many years to develop their skills. Their first operations are hardly as proficient as those that follow. Teaching with patients involves delays, diffusion of responsibility and accountability, and discomfort and even physical risk for the patient. Society permits these invasions of privacy and the risks attached to them not primarily so that physicians can make a living, but because society needs an uninterrupted supply of doctors. Medical knowledge and, analogously, legal and clerical knowledge, are held in trust for those who need them. These can never be dispensed solely for the profit of professionals or on terms unilaterally set by them. That is why lawyers are officers of the court, and clergy are ordained to minister in the name of God or of their churches.

The fifth feature of the professional relationship is that the professional is the **final common pathway** through which help and harm must pass. The final decisions, actions, and recommendations must be made by one person, the professional, with whom the patient or client has a conventional relationship of trust. No policy, no law, no regulation can be effective unless the physician, lawyer, or pastor permits it to influence the professional relationship. Professionals are allowed wide discretion because the needs of those they serve are unique. Professionals are thus guardians of the patient's interest and responsible for any act in which they participate.

The sixth distinguishing characteristic of professional relationships is that the professional is a member of **a moral community**, that is, a collective human association whose members share the privileges of special knowledge and together pledge their dedication to use it to advance health, justice, or salvation. Together the members of the moral community make the same promises and elicit the same trust that they do as individuals. They are bound by the same fidelity to the promise they have collectively made and the trust they have collectively elicited. The professional is therefore not a moral island. He belongs to a group that has been given a monopoly on special knowledge and holds it in trust for all who need it. Each professional is responsible to his colleagues, and they together are responsible for him. Collectively they are responsible for fidelity to the trust they have solicited from society. This is what the privilege of self-regulation means—that each professional is his own judge of what is ethically permissible.

These characteristics of human relationships are the components of the internal morality of the professions, the immediate moral ground for their obligations, and the source of definition of their virtues. To use Aristotle's terminology, these virtues make the work of the professions "be well done." The virtues of professional life are many, but they are reducible primarily to two—**fidelity to trust** and **beneficence**—which follow from the virtue of fidelity to trust. These two traits of character are the ethical foundations upon which the other virtues and principles of professional ethics depend. Clearly, they are incompatible with the Machiavellian and Hobbesian doctrines of self-interest. Their reality and irreducibility provide the most powerful argument for the restoration of virtue ethics in professional morality.[31]

The Practical Implications of Virtue Ethics: Self-Effacement

If there is validity in the philosophical foundations of professional morality, a number of practical implications follow that are pertinent to healing the moral malaise and confusion of today's professionals.

First, professionals cannot displace the moral failings of the professions onto others—on society, other professions, government, economics, the marketplace, and so on. No one can make the conscientious professional do what she thinks is not in the interests of the patient or client. Can anyone force doctors to follow a policy damaging to their interests? The fact that the professional is the final common pathway for all policies, decisions, and actions forces her to be the guardian of the interests of her patient or client. Indeed, she invited that responsibility when she invited the patient or client to trust her.

As a result, individual practitioners must be very careful in exonerating themselves from morally dubious practices on the basis of survival. Professional ethics will have no future if it is gradually suffocated by the moral compromises of individual professionals. There will be times when, as guardians of patients' welfare, physicians will have a moral obligation to refuse: they will refuse to "dump" the patient who cannot pay; they will refuse to discharge the patient before he is ready; they will refuse to act as society's fiscal agents; they will refuse to be seduced by the profits of investments and ownership of health facilities or bonuses for denying or delaying needed care; they will refuse to be gatekeepers, except to protect their patients from unnecessary medical interventions or procedures.[32] The physician of character will be the one who can reliably be expected to exhibit the virtues of fidelity to trust and effacement of self-interest.[33]

The second practical implication is that the individual professional must not be expected to stand by when the well-being of his patient or client is threatened. It is an obligation of the professions as moral communities to be advocates for those they serve, and to take collective action to ensure that their services are available and accessible to all, to protect those in need of healing, justice or salvation against legislation, and public or institutional policies that may harm them. The professions as moral communities must also take the responsibility for each member's ethical behavior seriously enough to monitor, discipline, and even remove each other when the canons of professional morality are violated. Think of the enormous moral power the professions could exert if they were truly the advocates of those they serve. Suppose that, in addition, all the helping professions were to combine their efforts. Could any society resist? Can they do less? In the face of this power, can any of the three great professions blame society for their own moral impotence at this time?[34]

A third implication is that the formation of character is as important in the education of professionals as their technical education. Although this was a major concern of professional education in the past, it has now been forsaken. Ever since Plato raised the question in the *Meno,* people have asked, can virtue be taught? We devote a subsequent chapter to this question. Obviously, the whole task of character formation cannot be left to the professional schools. Families, churches, and schools all shape students' character long before they enter professional schools. But these schools must also teach what it is to be a good physician, lawyer, or clergyperson—what kind of person the good professional ought to be. Much can be done in character formation when a student is motivated by the desire to be a good professional even if his education prior to entering medical school, law school, or the seminary was morally neutral or deficient.

The most effective instruments of character formation are the professionals who teach in medical and law schools and seminaries. But they must be able to demonstrate that competence and character are inseparable, and that fidelity to trust and self-effacement can be, and must be, indispensable traits of the authentic profession. Unfortunately, not enough professional school faculty members are convinced of this or are morally equipped to serve as models of virtue.

Paradigm cases of ethically sensitive professionals drawn from the history and tradition of each profession are also helpful. They are more effective than is generally realized. One of the tragedies of medical history is its depreciation of the lives of the great physicians. While biographies may not have much fascination for sophisticated medical historians, they still have inspirational value for the aspirants to medicine. Other professions have their morally paradigmatic biographies as well. Most professional students enter with some ideal of service in mind that the professional school has a responsibility to reinforce.

A fourth implication is that cure of the moral malaise of the professions requires more than reordering the social organization or tailoring the semantic and semiotic feature of professional codes, as Kultgen rather naively supposes.[35] What failings there are in the professions are failings in character and not in the language of our codes. If character and virtue are restored, the appropriate social reorganizations will follow—not the other way around.

Finally, there are theoretical reasons for a restoration of virtue, both in general and in professional ethics. Happily, a renaissance of interest among moral philosophers in this subject is very much in evidence. But virtue ethics must not be seen as self-sufficient or as antithetical to principle for duty-based systems of the analysis of ethical dilemmas. The theoretical challenge is to develop the logical connections between analytical and virtue ethics, between principles and character; to close the gap between cognition of the right and good and the motivation to do it; and finally, in the light of our whole analysis, to strike the morally defensible balance between self-interest and its effacement that recognizes the primacy of altruistic beneficence.

The theoretical challenges will be complicated because virtue- and duty-based ethics are today isolated from a more comprehensive moral philosophy that could tell us why we must be moral and what we define as the moral life. We need to reconnect ethics to some notion of the good and to a coherent philosophical anthropology. To this end, it might be well to reexamine the classical-medieval synthesis before ethics was torn form its roots in moral philosophy. That synthesis, amplified by our newer knowledge of human nature, derived from the biological and social sciences, and reflected upon theologically, might provide the new resuscitation that an effective virtue ethics demands.

For the time being, a reflection on the nature of professional relationships can be fruitful even in the absence of a comprehensive moral philosophy of which it might be a part. The internal morality of the professions, based on the realities of professional relationships, is clear enough to help us repair the ozone hole opened in the fabric of professional ethics, even if we cannot repair the whole moral atmosphere on which our society depends for its survival.

Conclusion

We have emphasized some of the elements common to the moral philosophy of the three professions of medicine, law, and the ministry. Many of these same features are shared by other professions. We would leave them to decide how the virtues of fidelity to trust and effacement of self-interest apply to them. Suppose that all the professions were to acknowledge virtue as a ground for moral accountability. Would this not be the leaven for raising the standards of conventional morality as well?

Notes

1. See the Address by S. Linowitz to the Cornell Law School (April 15, 1988). This speech by a distinguished lawyer details some of the ethical lapses at the moral margin in current legal practice.
2. J. Ladd, "The Internal Morality of Medicine. An Essential Dimension of the Patient-Physician Relationship," *The Clinical Encounter: The Moral Fabric of the Patient-Physician Relationship,* ed. E. E. Shelp (Dordrecht/Boston: D. Reidel, 1983), pp. 209–230.
3. Aristotle, *Nichomachean Ethics,* Bk. 9, c. 8, 1168–1169. In this chapter, Aristotle distinguishes two types of self-love: reproachful and virtuous. Reproachful self-love is self-love that arises not according to a rational principle but according to passion. The person who loves the self in this way desires what is advantageous, not what is noble. Idem. at 1169 4–6. The person of reproachful self-love assigns to himself the greater share of wealth, honor, and bodily pleasure. The person who demonstrates virtuous self-love is inspired by the rational principle to secure for the self the most noble goods. The actions of this person will benefit both himself and others.
4. Plato, *The Republic* 338C, trans. Richard W. Sterling and William C. Scott, (New York: Norton, 1985).
5. William K. C. Guthrie, *The Sophists* (London: Cambridge University Press, 1971). This is a thorough and detailed examination of the idea of self-interest and its relationship to justice in *The Republic.* It is particularly helpful in its discussion of how Hobbesian and Machiavellian strains were prefigured in the thinking of the Sophists.
6. Aristotle, supra note 2, Bk. 9, c. 8.
7. See John M. Cooper, *Reason and Human Good in Aristotle* (Cambridge, MA: Harvard University Press, 1975), for a consideration of Aristotle's view on love of self and of others.
8. Aristotle, supra note 2, 1155b, 31, 11568 9–10, 1159a 8–12, 28–33. See also William F. R. Hardie, *Aristotle's Ethical Theory* (Oxford: Clarendon Press, 1968), p. 326.
9. See Troels Engberg-Pedersen, *Aristotle's Theory of Moral Insight* (New York: Oxford University Press, 1983), pp. 237–262, for a penetrating analysis of *Eudeman Ethics,* Bks. 8 and 9.
10. Hardie, supra note 8, says that for Aristotle, "The end of the state is 'greater and more perfect' than the end of the individual" and thus, the activities of the statesman are aimed at happiness "for himself and his fellow citizens." Idem. at 216.
11. Plato, supra note 4, at 341c–347a.

12. See Cicero, *De Officiis*, Bk. 3, Ch. 13, trans. Walter Miller, (London: W. Heinemann, 1913).

13. See "Oath of Hippocrates," *Encyclopedia of Bioethics*, vol. 4, ed. Warren T. Reich (New York: Free Press, 1978), p. 1731.

14. Niccolo Machiavelli, *The Prince:* "[the prince] will find that some of the things that appear to be virtues will, if he practices them, ruin him, and some of the things that appear to be wicked will bring him security and prosperity." (Niccolo Machiavelli, *The Prince*, trans. with Introduction by George Bull [New York: Penguin Books, 1975], p. 92).

15. Bernard Mandeville, *The Fable of the Bees*, ed. with intro. by Phillip Harth (Harmondsworth: Penguin Books, 1970).

16. Friedrich W. Nietzsche, *On the Genealogy of Morals*, trans. Walter Kaufmann and R. J. Hollingdale (New York: Vintage Books, 1967).

17. Ayn Rand, *The Fountainhead* (New York: New American Library, 1971).

18. Thomas Hobbes, *Leviathan*, ed. Charles B. MacPherson (Harmondsworth: Penguin Books, 1985); see also Henry Sidgwick, *Outlines of the History of Ethics* (Boston: Beacon Press, 1960). Sidgwick neatly summarizes Hobbes' paradoxical view of social duty: "a view of social duty in which the only fixed positions were selfishness everywhere and unlimited power somewhere could not but appear offensively paradoxical."

19. See John Stuart Mill, chap. II, *Utilitarianism*, ed. George Sher (Indianapolis: Hackett, 1979).

20. Henry More, *Enchiridion Ethicum; the English Translation of 1690 Reproduced from the First Edition*, trans. Edward Southwell (New York: The Facsimile Text Society, 1930).

21. Joseph Butler, *Sermons* (Oxford: Clarendon Press, 1897).

22. Edmund L. Pincoffs, *Quandaries and Virtues: Against Reductivism in Ethics* (Lawrence: University Press of Kansas, 1986).

23. Edward O. Wilson, *Sociobiology, The New Synthesis* (Cambridge, MA: Belknap Press of Harvard University Press, 1975).

24. Thomas Nagel, *The Possibility of Altruism* (Princeton, NJ: Princeton University Press, 1978).

25. Philippa Poot, *Virtues and Vices and Other Essays in Moral Philosophy* (Berkeley: University of California Press, 1978).

26. G. E. M. Anscombe, "Modern Moral Philosophy," *Philosophy* 33(1) (Jan., 1958):1–19.

27. Alasdair C. MacIntyre, *After Virtue; A Study in Moral Theory*, 2d ed. (Notre Dame, IN: Notre Dame University Press, 1984).

28. Wilson, *Sociobiology*.

29. See generally Edmund D. Pellegrino, "What Is a Profession? The Ethical Implications of the F.T.C. Order and Some Supreme Court Decisions," *Survey of Ophthalmology* 29(3) (November-December 1984):1–15.

30. See Robert E. Goodin, *Protecting the Vulnerable: A Reanalysis of Our Social Responsibilities* (Chicago: University of Chicago Press, 1985). This author proposes vulnerability as a source of moral obligation in his analysis of our social responsibilities.

31. See Edmund D. Pellegrino and David C. Thomasma, *For the Patient's Good: The Restoration of Beneficence in Health Care* (New York: Oxford University Press, 1988).

32. See S. Ansberry, "Dumping the Poor," *Wall Street Journal* (November 29, 1988): 1.

33. H. Tristram Engelhardt and Michael E. Rie, "Morality for the Medical-Industrial Complex—A Code of Ethics for the Mass Marketing of Health Care," *The New England Journal of Medicine* 319(16) (October 20, 1988):1086–1089. These authors argue against

the thesis that we are presenting, particularly in their view that traditional standards must be tailored to conform to institutional and third-party payers' requirements.

34. Joan C. Callahan, *Ethical Issues in the Professional Life* (New York: Oxford University Press, 1988). This is an anthology dealing with the relationships between professional and ordinary morality, with contributions by philosophers and professionals in law, medicine, and business.

35. John H. Kultgen, *Ethics and Professionalism* (Philadelphia: University of Pennsylvania Press, 1988).

III

THE PRACTICE OF VIRTUE

13

How Does Virtue Make a Difference?

Kant said that "purity of heart is to will one thing." It may seem odd to quote the father of deontology at the start of a chapter devoted to the ways in which virtue ethics make a difference in the moral life of medicine, yet Kant's insight goes straight to the point. Without principles, the moral life would rest on sand. There is too much variability in modern, secular, pluralistic society to trust that every person would act virtuously, or even that we could agree on what virtuous activity would entail in such an environment. Yet the obverse is also true. Ethics is far more than obeying rules. In the most extreme form of a rule-based ethics, presumably, individuals need not accept the truth of the rules, just obey them. If the rules are obeyed, social conformity is achieved, but at the enormous cost of diminishing persons. This is a reductionistic ethic that relies on one virtue, obedience to the rules, to maintain the social order. It neglects all the other important virtues that enhance individual self-fulfillment and character.

In this chapter, we shall explore in more direct fashion some issues that we have touched on only tangentially in previous chapters. Our aim is to demonstrate how virtue ethics in medicine would make a difference in moral analysis and in the kinds of moral choices the agent makes in concrete cases.

We will contend that virtue-based ethics does, in fact, entail differences in the degree and kind of moral behavior from what fidelity to duty or principle may require. These differences are located in three features intrinsic to virtue ethics. The first is the concept of pursuit of excellence in the moral life, which the term *areté* implies from the beginning. While rarely fully realized, this drive to seek excellence grounds the two other features of virtue-based ethics that set it apart— its purity of intention and its sensitivity to moral complicity.

Let us examine first the question of moral excellence and its relationship to supererogation, which naturally comes to mind when we speak of excellence going beyond duty and principle.

Areté, Virtues, and Supererogation

Those who do not reject virtue ethics outright nonetheless remain skeptical that it differs in any substantive way from duty- or principle-based ethics when it comes to the resolution of a moral dilemma. If it is argued, as we do, that there is a difference in moral responsiveness, the objection is usually made that we are confusing virtue with supererogation. This is equally true of deontologists and consequentialists. The former, like Kant, would identify the virtuous person as one who does her duty in accord with the categorical imperative for duty's sake; the latter as one who fulfills the duty of acting always in accord with the principle of utility to maximize happiness. If, as we have argued, principles are essential to any integrated ethic of medicine, what and how does virtue-based ethics add to what principle- and duty-based ethics already require?

Are the differences that virtue-based ethics entails for the moral decisions we make simply examples of supererogatory acts—those that, by definition, are outside or beyond duty? Kant would say so, since a fundamental tenet of his moral philosophy is that moral worth attaches only to acts that must be done out of duty. That is why Kant equates virtue with doing one's duty and specific virtues with specific duties. This is the view with which contemporary philosophers—Feinberg, Urmson, and others—disagree only in that they assign moral worth to supererogatory acts even though they are, by definition, beyond duty.[1]

We do not see duty, nonduty, and beyond duty as three sharply demarcated regions of moral worth. Rather, they are points on a continuum, with an ideal of perfection at one end—the saint, perhaps—and the idea of the amoral sociopath at the other. In between, there are duties peculiar to us in the roles we play and duties we accept if we seek a moral life that aims for a closer approach to the ideal.

In this view, virtuous persons are distinguished as agents, and their acts as well, by a capacity to be disposed habitually not only to do what is required as duty but to seek the perfection—the excellence, the *areté* of a particular virtue. Virtuous persons, on the thesis we are expounding, see themselves as bound to act as excellently as possible in achieving their ends. For the physician, that end is the healing of the patient. The physician accepts as a duty what others do not require of themselves, thereby redefining the threshold between duty and supererogation.

This has some resemblance to De Nicola's view of morality as an art form—that is, it is more than a matter of following rules or principles mechanically. Supererogation leaves room for creativity in the moral life. De Nicola says, "This art is manifested in spontaneous and unselfconscious moral acts that exemplify character in rich and striking ways."[2]

The virtuous person is impelled by his virtues to strive for perfection—not because it is a duty, but because he seeks perfection in pursuit of the *telos* of whatever it is he is engaged in. He cannot act otherwise. It is part of his character. He is disposed habitually to fill out the potential for moral perfection inherent in his actions because he wishes to be as close to perfection as possible—to approach it asymptotically—realizing all the while that he cannot get there and, in that realization, being prevented from the vices of self-righteousness and hubris.

Taking this threshold concept into account, the virtuous person is one who places the point of separation between moral acceptability and moral unacceptability of a decision to act at a different place than would one who acts solely from principle, rule, or duty. The virtuous person will interpret the span of duty, principle, or rule more inclusively and more in the direction of perfection of the good end to which the action is naturally oriented.

Rights and Good Intention

For many ethicists today—both consequentialists and non-Kantian deontologists—the moral agent's intentions are irrelevant to the morality of a decision to act. The act itself or its consequences are the determinants of moral quality. Intention may be an indication of *character,* but it is the deed's conformity to duty or principle that counts, not the agent's intention, because good intentions may result in bad acts and vice versa. The reverse is the case for Kantian deontologists, for whom purity of intention is of the utmost importance; the decision to act must be based on a duty that one must intend for fulfill for its own sake and not for some other reason. An even more central place was given to intentionality by Abailard, for whom the morality of an act was entirely dependent upon good intention.[3]

Several recent moral philosophers, like Gewirth, Mackie, and Fried, have reaffirmed the place of intention in ethics.[4] While their views diverge from those of Thomas Aquinas, they are not in total dissonance with him. We regard Aquinas' viewpoint as still the richest, most insightful, and most morally relevant account of intentionality. We shall draw upon it for our depiction of the way the intentions of the virtuous person distinguish the choices she makes.

Intention in a formal sense is, as Fried puts it, the answer to the question "Why did you do that?"[5] Our intention reveals the purpose, reason, or design behind our pursuit of a particular end. Intentionality is a mark of our rationality, of our capacity to premeditate and act with a plan by which we select certain means that most expeditiously will attain the end we choose. Intention is an act of will that desires a certain end. But it is not necessarily the same as desire because we may desire something that we do not intend or act to bring about; for example, we might desire the death of a dear friend who is suffering, but we do not will to act to achieve it. By contrast, we may intend something we do not desire, such as risking an operation or entering a battle.

Intention plays a significant role in the moral quality of our acts because it reveals the kinds of persons we are, that is, the character we possess. Our acts may produce a good result—like giving alms—but if our intent in giving alms is to enhance our reputations or to escape paying income tax, then what could be good loses moral merit by the imperfection of our intention. Conversely, a good intention cannot make an act morally good. Some species of acts, like adultery, or torture, or killing the innocent, are wrong as a species.

The virtuous person exhibits as close a congruence as possible between the interior and exterior dimensions of moral acts. Her intent is moral excellence, and she strives to choose means to that end that themselves are as excellent as the circumstances will allow.

The virtuous physician will intend means that will be most perfectly in the best interests of the sick person. She will act in the patient's best interests because that is what the end of medicine and the covenant of trust between doctor and patient imply that she ought to do. She will be faithful to this trust not because she fears a malpractice suit, or because it is good for her reputation, or will bring the patient back for another visit, or will result in a referral of another patient. Excellence of intent is not self-righteous—it does not compare itself to others, to its own advantage, or follow moral rules so as to be morally "one up." Excellence in medical intent requires the possession of virtues that will enable the good intention—that is, one focused on the good of the patient—to be actualized by the physician's behavior.

Moral Complicity

Intention centers on freely willed acts the effects of which we foresee. We are not morally responsible for harmful effects we do not foresee. But there is a large category of acts in which, by dint of circumstances, both good and harmful effects may ensue. These are accidental effects. While we do not intend the attendant harm, we may be moral accomplices. The degree of our complicity depends upon the foreseeable possibility, probability, and avoidability of the "accidents." This is especially the case in the use of medical knowledge that may have both beneficial and harmful effects, proximate or ultimate.

At some time, perhaps even as a matter of course in certain medical occupations (e.g., physicians in prisons, penal institutions, mental hospitals, or military service), physicians may find themselves in situations in which law, social conventions, or institutional policies conflict with the primary orientation of medicine to the good of the person who is ill or in need of help.[6] In these instances, physicians are in socially legitimated and even necessary roles, acting simultaneously as physicians and as agents of institutional purpose.

The situations in which possible complicity with what is morally wrong or dubious are many. They range from the grossly immoral to the morally dubious—from direct participation in the torture of political prisoners, to testifying in a psychiatric commitment proceeding, to the conflicts-of-interest involved in self-referral. In all of these instances, the primary end of the welfare of the sick person is distorted or displaced in varying degrees by economic, political, legal, or selfish motives. Society may legitimate various occupations in this spectrum of complicity, but health professionals cannot dissociate themselves from the harm or danger to the patient that may result from well-intentioned cooperation.

When it comes to the use of medical knowledge, the physician or nurse is the agent through whom society and institutions must operate. It is the health professional who writes or carries out medical orders. It is her expertise that is essential to the purposes to which the state or institution wishes to put medical knowledge.

This is not the place to set out the criterion by which licit or illicit cooperation may be determined. One of us (EDP) has done so elsewhere.[7] What is relevant here is the fact that a physician operating within the framework of virtue-based ethics will habitually, predictably, and sensitively ascertain what is a morally acceptable degree of cooperation and what is not. Here the virtue of prudence is particularly relevant. It enables the physician to discern what degree of cooperation balances the conflicting obligations in the most judicious way. Prudence is the early warning device against morally intolerable cooperation with evil.

Some Practical Decisions in the Light of Virtue Ethics

The differences between duty- and principle-based ethics and virtue ethics are most manifest at the moral margin, in those regions of the moral life where law, custom, or principle would allow certain acts (or fail to prohibit them) that virtue would prohibit. Several concrete examples drawn from the practical sphere will serve to illustrate the differences we have been discussing. These differences are the results of the practice of specific virtues we have examined in earlier chapters.

Models of the Physician–Patient Relationship

Currently, the nature of the physician–patient relationship, like every other facet of professional ethics, is under critical scrutiny. The traditional notion of a **covenant of trust** in which the physician ensures competence that will be used for the patients well-being is being challenged by a series of alternate models. Some suggest that the relationship is more realistically approached as a **contract**; others, as a **free market relationship**, with physician as supplier and patient as consumer; still others see the physician primarily as a **mechanic**, technician, teacher, social servant, educator, and advisor, but primarily as an instrument of the patient's autonomy.

Each model generates different duties and is guided by different principles. Depending on the strength of the arguments marshaled, none inherently is excluded by principle- or duty-based ethics. To be sure, the medical relationship has elements of all of these models in some measure. The question, however, is, which should be predominant?

In an ethic that strives for excellence in moral life, one exemplified by practice of the virtues we have outlined in this book, certain of the alternate models would simply be inconceivable. Virtue-based ethics is not compatible with a **contract** model, which, like a legal contract, presumes that the interacting agents are equal bargainers. Contracts are based on an assumption of mistrust that requires obligations to be spelled out in detail. Contracts are not instruments of beneficence. They are minimalistic, legalistic, and subject to disputes over performance. A contract model obliges the physician only to perform what is spelled out. Fidelity to a contract is a duty, but it is insufficient if moral excellence is a goal.

Similar objections are built into the **consumer–producer model**, in which the ethos of the marketplace predominates. This model legitimates the physician's role as primarily that of a businessperson or entrepreneur. Competence is assured for fear of malpractice. Compassion, trust, benevolence, and even justice inevitably come into competition with the economic self-interest of the physician as entrepreneur. The marketplace is not driven by ethical but rather by economic forces. Health care cannot be a commodity whose distribution, price, quality, or availability can be left to the forces of competition. Effacement of self-interest is antithetical to this model. Virtue, if practiced, is practiced only because it is also "good business."

The other alternate models have their own deficiencies when viewed from the standpoint of an ethic that seeks moral excellence. The model of the physician as a **mechanic** makes competence the predominant virtue; caring models put compassion in that position; and hieratic models grant quasi-religious authority to physicians. Each model reduces duty or principle to one facet of the relationship. Each facet defines a different end for medicine and, if pursued to any degree of excellence, can distort **the healing relationship**. The virtuous physician oriented to the excellence of the moral life in medicine is disposed to a more comprehensive view of its ends, one that considers the whole good of the patient.

Care of the Poor

While *pro bono* work is encouraged by traditional ethics of medicine, it is not a widely imposed duty or principle. The Hippocratic ethic is unclear on the extent to which care of the poor is an obligation. For the virtuous physician in pursuit of excellence in the moral life, medical knowledge, however, is not proprietary. It is held in stewardship for those who need it and not just for those who can pay. All who are sick have a claim to medical knowledge. Virtue-based ethics would respond to that claim on the part of individual physicians and the whole medical community. A virtuous profession would provide the support of the medical community for the virtue of solicitude for the impoverished sick.

Care of the Noncompliant and the Self-Abuser

There is a growing sentiment in the public and the profession that some persons are not worthy of health care or use up their entitlement because of their behavior. This category includes patients who refuse or fail to follow the physician's orders, who abuse alcohol or drugs, or who routinely fail to observe reducing diets, to give up smoking, or to take medication regularly. Some argue that, given the scarcity of health care resources and the cost of health care, there is an obligation to conserve society's resources by refusing to treat such patients. Others, at a minimum, see no obligation to treat them.

Physicians motivated by virtue would reject such propositions. Whatever the patient's moral failings or foibles, they would feel constrained to treat those in need of their help as best as they can without moralizing and without self-righteous or retributive attitudes. This does not suggest approval of self-abusive or noncompliant behavior. Nor does it suggest abandonment of efforts to change the patient's behavior. Similar nondiscriminatory, nonretaliative attitudes would be taken with respect to patients with HIV infection, patients who are considered "difficult" or unworthy, or patients with venereal or contagious diseases.

Managed Health Care

Various forms of organized medical practice have appeared of late, many of which pose direct challenges to the primacy of patient welfare by putting the physician in a position of double agency—simultaneously serving the patient, and the institutional policy. Whether the motive is making a profit, keeping costs down by cutting corners diagnostically or therapeutically, refusing to see patients without adequate insurance, effecting the "economic transfer" of indigent patients, or applying policies designed primarily to protect the institution, the potential for compromising the patient's welfare is a genuine danger. Often these practices are rationalized—and even made matters of duty claims—on the basis of fiscal exigency or operational efficacy.

All of these arrangements, to some degree, distort the ends of medicine and impel the virtuous physician to avoid complicity by avoiding such arrangements. Where participation is unavoidable because of circumstances, virtue ethics requires the physician to minimize the compromise of patient welfare. Where the harm is grave, she must resist and refuse to comply. As a moral community, the organized profession should support the physicians who will not compromise the primacy of patient welfare.

In the case of penal, military, or forensic medicine, "double agency" is a matter of daily course. Physicians so employed should make their "double agency" abundantly clear so that patients or those they attend will not be deceived into believing that they are in a normal physician–patient relationship. If certain constraints on moral complicity are observed, the virtuous physician can serve in these "dual agency" roles.[8]

Conflicts of Interest: For-Profit Service

The increasing commercialization and industrialization of medicine and medical care create opportunities for personal profit to physicians that are increasingly legitimated, often under the illusion that they will reduce health care costs. Ownership of laboratories, nursing homes, and imaging centers, pharmacies, office dispensing of drugs, and a variety of emoluments are now widely available to practitioners and academicians alike. These emoluments begin with medical students. Medical schools, clinical investigators, and basic scientists in this era of cooperative research have much to gain financially by close relationships with the pharmaceutical or medical appliance industries. Many of these arrangements are considered morally licit, not inconsistent with duty- or principle-based ethics, and even commendable.

However, without impugning the motives of the physicians and institutions now enjoying these arrangements or the good things that may result, there remains the inescapable human inclination to compromise integrity in the cause of self-interest. As a result, scientific data, research protocols, the context of scientific or technical consultations, and the management of patients in clinical investigation may subtly be or overtly shaped to please the funding source. Physicians who follow a virtue-based ethic would avoid most of these practices—at least those in which the potential for compromise or scientific integrity of patient welfare is a real possibility. This is a moral realm in which the temptation to self-delusion and self-justification is strong, as anyone will attest who has tried to fashion a conflict-of-interest policy for either practitioners or academicians.

Clearly, our view of the virtues would extend them beyond the limits of the morally obligatory, that is, beyond duties into the realm of the supererogatory. Many will object that the very term "supererogatory" takes an act out of the realm of duty. Strictly by definition, this is so. But this does not allow for the fact that we all recognize grades of commendability in moral actions. Some persons seem in their actions to come closer to the spirit behind the principle and to appreciate its finer nuances. They go somewhat beyond what others might think obligatory—even those who accept the same principle. They take a principle of morality to higher gradations of congruence and so fulfill more of what a principle implies.

There is a moral realm somewhere between supererogation of a heroic kind (e.g., giving one's whole life to the care of the most deprived, like Mother Theresa) and mechanically fulfilling the requirements of moral principles, as Hare puts it, like "copybook headings" or as a way to "avoid doing any more thinking about particular cases."[9] Between these extremes are those persons we call "good" or "superior" persons, doctors, lawyers, pastors, or parents. They are not saints or heroes, but they represent a degree of virtue we admire because it is more than the minimum required by mere conforming to principle or duty.

The virtues, thus, give an added dimension to moral principle. This is important when the moral standards of a society are minimal or eroding. In a society in which effacement of self-interest is losing ground to self-interest, self-effacement tends to become supererogatory. But in certain activities, like medicine, what is supererogatory in general society may be morally obligatory. The person of virtue, and the physician who cultivates the virtues entailed in the ends of medicine, will recognize this difference. This, at times, will require the additional virtue of courage to persist in acting against those general moral trends in society that are inimical to medical ethics.

Frankena nicely captures some of the nuances of the relationship of principle and virtue in his "parody" of Kant: "Principle without traits are impotent, traits without principles are blind."[10] Virtue- and principle-based ethics need each other. But we would go further and say that virtue gives something more than another perspective. Possessing a virtue, as Bernard Williams avers, "affects how one deliberates."[11] Certain options in moral choice are simply, on the face of it, not acceptable and not options to a virtuous person.

In medical ethics we see the virtues as disposing physicians and nurses to higher degrees of sensitivity to self-determination, fidelity to trust, intellectual honesty, benevolence, and justice because these virtues are integral to attaining the ends of the practice of medicine. These virtues are not simply skills, but essential traits if the good of patients is to be furthered optimally by our medical actions. The virtues are essential in medicine because the phenomenology of illness and healing is not fully comprehensible as a moral challenge by principles alone. The virtues enable us asymptotically to approach the fullness of the yearning to heal.

Conclusion

In this investigation we have tried to show, using a few examples, that virtue ethics does make a difference in the realm of practical decisions. According to the ethic of virtue, physicians who strive for excellence in the medical moral life will, by definition, be more sensitive to their inner intentions and the possibility of moral complicity. They will be more likely to locate the dividing line between what is morally licit and what is illicit at a different place than duty- or principle-based ethics would require.

Whether this is supererogation is not morally crucial. To raise the question is really to beg the question, since supererogation, by definition, means "beyond duty." We have argued that virtue-based ethics does, in one sense, go beyond duty. In another sense, which we favor, virtue-based ethics stays within the realm of principle and duty. But it pursues moral excellence in the performance of duties or adherence to principles.

Certainly, the profession should emphasize fidelity to duty and principle. These are the foundational beginnings of the moral life. But they are not its full substance. Without some core of physicians who live according to the spirit of a virtue ethic, the profession is not likely to achieve the fullness of its potential as a force for human good. Nor will it serve its constituency as a safeguard against the deterioration of moral standards and principles to which any society may be, at times, susceptible. We must not forget that the interpretation of principles and their hierarchical ordering may change. Virtues, on the other hand, interpreted as we have suggested in terms of the healing intent of medicine, are less susceptible to such change.

Principles and duties are the letter of medical ethics. It remains to virtue to live according to the spirit of medical ethics, which has been and should remain focused on the good of the sick person. Principles and duties enable physicians to do good, but virtues enable them to be good, to make the difference that can make a competent professional a noble one.

Notes

1. Daniel R. De Nicola, "Supererogation, Artistry in Conduct," *Issues in Philosophical Ethics*, ed. LeRoy S. Rouner (Notre Dame, IN: University of Notre Dame Press, 1983), pp. 155–159. Also see Gregory Mellema, *Beyond the Call of Duty: Supererogation, Obligation, and Offence* (Albany, N.Y.: State University of New York Press, 1991); David Heyd, *Supererogation: Its Status in Ethical Theory* (New York: Cambridge University Press, 1982).

2. Ibid., p. 162.

3. Abailard, *Abailard's Ethics*, trans. and intro. by J. Ramsay MaCallum (Merrick, NY: Richwood, 1976).

4. Alan Gewirth, *Reason and Morality* (Chicago: University of Chicago Press, 1978); J. L. Mackie, *Ethics: Inventing Right and Wrong* (New York: Penguin Books, 1978); Charles Fried, *Right and Wrong* (Cambridge, MA: Harvard University Press, 1978).

5. Fried, *Right and Wrong,* pp. 24–28.

6. Edmund D. Pellegrino, "Cooperation, Moral Complicity, and Moral Distance: The Ethics of Forensic, Penal, and Military Medicine," *International Journal of Law and Psychiatry* (in press).

7. Ibid.

8. Ibid.

9. R. M. Hare, *Freedom and Reason,* (New York: Oxford University Press, 1965), p. 37.

10. William Frankena, *Ethics,* 2d ed. (Englewood Cliffs, NJ: Prentice-Hall, 1973), p. 53.

11. Bernard Williams, *Ethics and the Limits of Philosophy* (Cambridge, MA: Harvard University Press, 1985), p. 10.

14

Can the Medical Virtues Be Taught?

Can you tell me, Socrates, is virtue something that can be taught? Or does it come by practice? Or is it neither teaching nor practice that gives it to a man, but natural aptitude or something else?

Meno

In his celebrated but characteristically indecisive dialogue with Meno, Socrates posed the question that still worries the critics and even the friends of ethics: Can good character be taught? More specifically for the purposes of this book, Can the virtues essential to the formation of the good physician be taught, and, if so, How?

To answer the question, as Socrates pointed out to Meno, we must know what virtue is and, then, by what method we should teach it. In this book, we have tried, with the post-Socratic insights provided by Aristotle, Aquinas, and other thinkers, to define virtue in general and then those individual virtues important to attaining the ends of medicine. We can now turn, with somewhat less assurance, to a qualified answer to Socrates' question. Yes, we think the virtues essential to being a good physician can be taught—at least in part, and with some hope of success.

The objections against our position are detailed powerfully in the *Meno*. There Socrates presents Meno with three cases of worthy men whose sons were not as virtuous as their fathers. He cites Themistocles, Aristides, and Pericles. These were men of virtue, yet they were not able to teach their virtues to the sons or to find anyone else who could do so. They could teach many other concepts and skills; why could they not teach virtue? At the end of the dialogue, with the caveat that the discourse is not finished until virtue can be defined, Socrates concludes that men learn virtue only by "divine inspiration."[1]

Anytus, who later urged at Socrates' trial that he be put to death, takes the opposite view. He is supremely confident that virtue can be taught and that all one has to do to learn is to observe "good" Athenians. Anytus is arguing that virtue can be taught by good example and good models.

Today's skeptics would side with Socrates' assertion that we do not know what virtue is, that it cannot be taught, and that character is inborn—or, at least, that it

175

is so fully developed by the time a person enters medical school that it is impossible to change it.

We cannot agree with Anytus' confident, indeed arrogant, assertion that "any decent Athenian gentleman"[2] can teach virtue. Nor can we agree with Socrates in the *Meno* that virtue is indefinable, that it cannot be taught, and that we are forced to believe in divine infusion of the virtues.

Rather, like Plato in *The Republic,* and like Aristotle, Aquinas, and Dewey, we believe that virtue can be taught by practice, by example, and even by the study of ethics. In making this assertion, we would be modest in our expectations but firm in our rejection of the futility of teaching virtue even in unpromising situations.

The Skeptical View of Teaching Medical Virtues

Let us begin by confronting the major objections leveled by today's skeptics:

First, it is argued that virtue is best taught by the school, family, and religious community—church, synagogue, or mosque. This is surely the case for most people. Medical students do arrive with certain well-established fundamental moral values when they enter medical school. Indeed, a survey by one of us[3] indicates that these values rarely are changed by courses in ethics.

But we must make a distinction here. What we can hope to teach in medical school are those virtues appropriate to medicine—those that make for a good physician judged in terms of the *telos* of medicine, that is, a right and good healing action for a particular patient. We do not propose that a medical school, especially in a pluralistic society, can alter fundamental religious beliefs or nonbeliefs. It is unavoidable that these received values will be reexamined by the medical school experience. The medical faculty cannot substitute for the home, church, or school. What that faculty can teach is what it is to be a good physician *qua* physician, and to practice and value the virtues requisite for good medicine as we have spelled them out in this book.

By emphasizing the virtues of the physician *qua* physician, we are not ignoring the importance of the virtues of the person as person. In subtle ways, the virtues of the good person and of the good physician overlap. Educating for virtue in one domain undoubtedly influences the other. But we will confine our examination to the formation of a good medical character, one built on the virtues of the physician *qua* physician.

If we accept this as the aim of virtue education proper to a medical school, then the argument that it is too late to teach virtue in medical school loses its force. Medical students come to medical school precisely for the purpose of being educated to be physicians. There is a relevance and an inevitability about this fact that make character education a *de facto* reality. Whether the faculty wishes it or not, they do teach virtue or vice in everything they say or do. This applies equally to basic scientists and clinicians.

Any physician at all reflective about his own education will admit the reality of models. Indeed, one of the most distinctive features of the profession is the way in which physicians honor their teachers, a residue of the Hippocratic tradition and, specifically, the preamble to the Oath.[4] The way each physician construes medicine, confronts the daily dilemmas of practice, or thinks about clinical decisions has been influenced by good and bad models. All physicians have encountered teachers they wish to emulate and others they would not wish to be associated with.

Usually, the student's initial attraction to a particular faculty model is through the proficiency of that model in her discipline. Understandably, the most influential models are in the field the student plans to enter. Excellent performance as a teacher, investigator, or clinician naturally stimulates the interest of students with some concept of what they would like to become professionally. The character traits of the faculty model are unconsciously imitated as well. Indeed, the faculty model's professional standing as a scientist or clinician often legitimates her personal ethical behavior as well. That behavior might be something the student previously had considered morally dubious or unacceptable.

Ruefully, medical school training is sometimes a breeding ground for aggressiveness, pride, poor communication with patients, and other character traits that directly contravene the virtues we have examined thus far. The standard criticisms of medical school training are built on this experience. Too often, previously altruistic students are subject to systematic pressure that undermines altruism and rewards selfishness and competition. Under the pressure to conform in order to succeed and not to imperil a career, even a virtuous student will need extra courage to resist.

The power of a faculty model to shape behavior for good or evil is enormous. It far exceeds the power of a lecture or courses in ethics. This power generates a serious *de facto* obligation for faculty members and medical schools to be critical of the value systems they express and transmit. Earlier we discussed the problem of whether or not institutions might be said to have a conscience or to be held accountable for their behaviors. Medical schools are a good example of such institutions. They do shape in fact the conduct of their faculty and students. They are responsible thereby for the values they teach. The challenge is to direct the molding process toward a virtuous mode of practicing medicine.

Academic freedom does not justify behavior that violates the canons of ethical science or medicine. One of the saddest aspects of professional ethics today is the frequency with which senior and respected teachers have perpetrated and justified such acts as conflicts-of-interest, fudging and selective reporting of data, insensitivity to patients' needs, inadequate consent for procedures—experimental or therapeutic—or toleration of incompetent colleagues. The long-term effects of such bad examples on the present and future generation of scientists and clinicians are incalculable.

Unfortunately, examples of morally dubious behavior abound. Many physicians today are lured into conflicts-of-interest by the funding they receive from drug companies or device manufacturers. They might surround their presentations with appropriate caveats, but their reputations and income often are too closely linked to certain procedures, methods, or medications.[5] Irresponsible reporting of data, inappropriate supervision of assistants, and outright fraud have been suspected and even discovered in major academic institutions and researchers. The Office of Scientific Integrity of the NIH came under fire by its own NIH director in 1991 when it released negative reports on the integrity of physicians in Baltimore, at the Cleveland Clinic, and in France on each of these points.[6] Later it was closed!

Some of the blame for these moral lapses is attributable to the way scientific research support is currently structured. But ultimately, it is the character of the researcher that stamps each scientific endeavor with its moral quality.[7]

These moral aberrations are not confined to medicine. Law, teaching, and the clergy all have been lax in maintaining their traditional ethical standards. Some practitioners have been jailed for bilking the public, making money on questionable research results, and violating the public trust by insider trading. All the professions, as a result, are suffering today a loss of public confidence and inviting external regulation to degrees that will limit their discretionary latitude and ultimately their capacity to act in the best interest of patients, clients, parishoners, or students.[8] Intelligence is not enough. Character and virtue must precede it in human affairs.

The tragic outcome of lax virtue is to invite increased societal control over the profession by means of externally imposed rules and regulations. These not only shrink professional latitude, as noted above, but also diminish the professional as a person. If virtue is not practiced, then external rules will govern the moral life. The virtues are not internalized, and the opportunity for moral growth by practice of the virtues is lost. The end result is a diminution of the human potential and fulfillment of the professional person.

In any case, the fact that students indeed are influenced by the ethical standards of their teachers, particularly their teachers' professional ethics, is proof enough that virtue and vice can be taught. Professional schools, as a result, have the responsibility to attend consciously to the content, ethical probity, and quality of such teaching.

This is a responsibility medical schools never have attended to as institutions. Yet society has at least implicit expectations that medical schools will provide some assurance of the characters of their graduates. Given the power to do harm and good that a medical degree confers on the students, one of us (Pellegrino) has argued that there is a communal responsibility of medical faculties to detect, at minimum, the most egregious character defects, and attempt to correct them.[9] Most medical students will state that they can readily recognize the members of their class whom they would not trust with their patients.[10] Yet most medical faculties are insufficiently acquainted with their students' behavior to make such judgments.

One might argue that the medical school has only one responsibility: to ensure satisfaction of the intellectual academic requirements for the degree. This, we hold, is insufficient. Teaching virtue is a responsibility grounded in the social mandate and the covenant a school enters into with society. If a school of divinity pays attention, as it should, to the spiritual formation of its future ministers, can the medical school ignore the character of its graduates? The answer seems to us to be that the essential moral nature of healing compels attempt to instill virtue as well as technical knowledge in medical students.[11] Again, to avoid confusion, we speak here of the virtues of the physician *qua* physician, not the virtues of the physician *qua* person, which is a broader and more private enterprise.

Teaching Ethics and the Role of Virtues

Though the best way to teach virtuous behavior is by example, some significant headway can be made by teaching ethics as a discipline.[12] To be sure, there is no guarantee that a knowledge of ethics itself will make people virtuous. The moral lapses of professional ethicists stand as proof of the lack of correlation between knowing the good and doing the good. However, teaching ethics as a discipline does sensitize students to what constitutes an ethical issue or problem. When properly taught, it forces self-criticism and examination of one's own values. It demands that reasons be given for moral choices, that opposing viewpoints be given an adequate response, and it encourages the laying bare of underlying prelogical assumptions in any ethical argument. If any of these end results are achieved, even in part, they cannot help but have some impact on the character of the student. For this reason, we have urged that ethics should be taught in medical schools as a regular part of the curriculum.[13]

A favorite rejoinder to those who argue that virtue can be taught is the evaluation gambit: how can you prove that your teaching has had an effect? The question is easier to answer for teaching ethics as a discipline than for teaching virtue. Here the teaching objective is knowledge of the technique of ethical analysis, or knowledge of competing ethical theories, the meaning of terms used in ethical discourse, and of the growing literature of ethical argument and practice as they relate to the day-by-day dilemmas of the medical encounter. These objectives can be examined objectively and, thus, measured in the same way as the effectiveness of teaching in any other discipline.[14]

When it comes to virtue, however, the end point is a change in human character, a strengthening of virtuous intention and practices, and a deepening of the disposition to do the morally right thing even when no one is watching. To test for this outcome, we would have to observe our subjects in a variety of moral situations before and after our attempts to teach virtue. The methodological difficulties of such a study are obviously insurmountable.

Do these difficulties render all attempts to teach virtue useless or pointless? We think not. There are many things we do in medical education that do not yield to easy measurement. Even those studies whose effectiveness we think we can measure are on similarly insecure ground. Do we know, for example, to what degree courses in the basic sciences make for better clinical decisions? Anyone who has taught some aspect of the basic sciences to students in the clinical years (as has EDP for many years) appreciates how insecure is the grasp of even pathophysiology by some very good clinicians. The uncertainty of evaluation notwithstanding, we would not argue that teaching physiology or molecular biology is useless for clinicians.

In any case, as we have suggested above, medical faculties cannot avoid teaching virtue or vice along with basic science and clinical medicine. As teachers, they cannot escape projecting their own moral values through their teaching. This being the case, regardless of whether the end results are measurable, there is a moral obligation to give a place to character in our teaching.

It is unescapably true that, at some point in every clinical encounter, the patient's final safety and well-being depend on the character of the physician. It is through the physician that all orders must pass. It is she who must cooperate with or resist policies and decisions that may affect a particular patient's well-being. The physician is often the final safeguard of the incompetent patient when economic, emotional, or selfish motives may becloud a surrogate's choices. Physicians cannot escape the **covenant of trust** implicit in **the healing relationship**. How sensitive they are to the implications of that covenant will depend upon the kinds of persons they have become. The moral agent and the moral act are indissolubly united in the moment of clinical decision.

Because of this indissolubility, like it or not, medical faculties have a *de facto* obligation to take some responsibility for character formation—at least insofar as acquisition of the virtues of the good physician are concerned. Faculties can fulfill this responsibility, first by example in the laboratory and at the bedside, then by teaching ethics as a discipline and assuming shared responsibility for the moral sensitivity of their students. The medical school and the profession are moral communities,[15] and moral consensus in those communities is essential if the practices of the virtuous physician are to be sustained.

This sense of a moral community requires appropriate action whenever there is sufficient evidence of a serious character flaw in a student or faculty member that might endanger the patient, society, and the scientific enterprise itself. We are not recommending a dogmatic, doctrinaire, or restrictive approach to medical education. Rather, what is needed is sensitivity and responsiveness to obvious morally aberrant behavior—something that unfortunately occurs in every environment. Too often patent dishonesty, scientific fraud, and incompetence are neglected or even covered over due to a mistaken notion of loyalty or because of pious promises of reform. Instead, the academic community should reinforce the behavior of its members who exhibit ethical sensitivity. We discussed this in Chapter 10.

Admissions Selection as a Technique to Promote Virtue

Picking students of good character is the hope of every medical school admissions committee. If the committee is successful, the school will have taken a major first step in producing virtuous physicians. But as we shall see, this is problematic.

If character and virtue are so essential to moral conduct in the physician–patient relationship, why not simplify matters by selecting students on the basis of character in the first place? This is an attractive idea, and it certainly would ameliorate the problem. Unfortunately, there is no reliable or practical way to assess an applicant's character.

Some suggest that the admissions interview is the best means. Like Anytus in the *Meno,* they are confident of their own ability to judge who will make a good doctor. Others would turn to letters from people they know to be reliable observers of human character. Others would administer psychological tests of attitude and of moral values. Still others would look for some records of public service. None of these methods is without value. However, each is subject to grave error and even to abuse that would pose the possibility of serious injustice to applicants, especially those outside the dominant social or ethnic group.

Interviewers, being human, tend to favor applicants with values most like their own. Character references notoriously are unreliable in this age of litigation. Psychological tests have large margins of error and are too easily "psyched out" by clever exam takers. Finally, how can we tell whether a record of community services was inspired by altruism or by the knowledge that it would impress an admission committee? Most often, medical school applicants have been thoroughly coached about what impresses the interviewers and the committee. In effect, all we might be selecting are individuals who know how to "interview well."

Clearly, admission committees should use all available sources bearing on an applicant's character. But on the whole, medical school classes will end up being representative of the values of American society, some of which are consistent with what is required of a good physician and some not. Given the powerful way in which the medical school's own moral climate can shape the image of the physician, our contention is that medical faculties must be concerned about the moral values they transmit to their students. Ideally, they would be cognizant of their own moral values and able to discuss these with their patients and their peers.[16]

To recognize the *de facto* teaching of character and the attendant responsibility of medical schools does not, however, absolve students from responsibility for moral lapses later in life. To blame the medical school for our own dishonesty, cheating, malpractice, competitiveness, or medical fraud is a moral "copout." Although they are powerful influences, medical schools offer only a time-limited experience. One fashions one's self-image as a physician over a whole lifetime. To blame our training for our vices is transparently disingenuous. At the worst, one might conceivably accuse a medical school of contributory negligence if it had knowingly graduated incompetent and/or psychopathic students.

Conclusion

We have focused on teaching virtue and character formation in medical school. What we have said applies with even more force to residency training and to the practice milieu. These are even more powerful influences. In residency training the contact with faculty models is very close, so that the temptation and pressure to conform are difficult to resist. Moreover, in residency, one has chosen a field with which one identifies. To "rock the boat" by not conforming even to distorted moral values is to alienate oneself and to imperil one's career.

These pressures are recognized by the major specialty boards, which lately have insisted on ethics training for their residents. Some of these training programs are designed ambitiously. For example, the American Board of Orthopedics, the American Board of Internal Medicine, and the American Board of Ophthalmology, just to name three, have rigorous requirements. We fear that they will be disappointed if they surmise that this exposure to ethics and the other humanities will guarantee a more virtuous practitioner of the art. After all, Reinhard Heydrich, one of the most vicious of all the Nazis, also was the most classically learned. He chaired the meeting in the suburb of Wansee that was to bring about "a complete solution of the Jewish question in the German sphere of influence in Europe."[17]

In practice, the pressure to conformity is even greater. It is more difficult to change the venue. What has become standard practice too often becomes right practice without any real inquiry into the moral status of that practice. In our last chapter, we address the implications of the professions as moral communities. Suffice it to say that education in character and virtue occurs throughout the life of a practitioner. Moral maturity, like professional competence, takes time, cultivation, and critical self-appraisal.

Notes

1. Plato, *Meno,* 70a 1–5.

2. Ibid., 92e.

3. Edmund D. Pellegrino and Thomas K. McElhinney, *Teaching Ethics, the Humanities, and Human Values in Medical Schools: A Ten Year Overview* (Washington, DC: Institute on Human Values in Medicine and the Society for Health and Human Values, 1982).

4. Hippocrates, *Oath in Hippocrates I,* Loeb Classic Library, trans. W. H. S. Jones (Cambridge, MA: Harvard University Press, 1962), p. 299.

5. Note the warnings about laser surgery in *Consumer Reports* (July 1991): 6–8.

6. See John Crewdson, *Column, Chicago Tribune* July 21, 1991, Sec. 1, 3; also *Chicago Tribune,* July 28, 1991, Sec. 1, 4; and *Chicago Tribune,* July 31, 1991, Sec. 1, 2.

7. Edmund D. Pellegrino, "Character and the Ethical Conduct of Research," *Accountability in Research* 2(1) (1992):1–12.

8. Thomas Jefferson to Peter Carr, August 1785, in Julian P. Boyd (ed.), *The Papers of Thomas Jefferson,* Vol. 8, ed. Julian P. Boyd (Princeton, NJ: Princeton University Press, 1953), p. 406.

9. Edmund D. Pellegrino, "The Medical Profession as a Moral Community," *Bulletin of the New York Academy of Medicine* 66(3) (May-June 1990):221–232.

10. Edmund D. Pellegrino, "Medical Education," *The Encyclopedia of Bioethics*, Vol. 2, ed. Warren T. Reich (New York: Free Press-Macmillan, 1978), pp. 863–870.

11. Edmund D. Pellegrino and David C. Thomasma, *Health and Healing,* (in press).

12. Edmund D. Pellegrino, "Teaching Medical Ethics: Some Persistent Questions and Some Responses," *Aademic Medicine: The Journal of the Association of American Medical Colleges* 64(12) (December 1989):701–703.

13. Pellegrino and McElhinney, *Ten Year Overview.*

14. Edmund D. Pellegrino, "Can Ethics Be Taught? An Essay," *Mt. Sinai Journal of Medicine* 56(6) (November 1989):490–494.

15. Pellegrino, "Medical Profession as Moral Community."

16. David C. Thomasma, and Patricia M. Marshall, "The Clinical Humanities Program at Loyola University of Chicago," *Academic Medicine* 64(12) (December 1989):735–739. The entire issue of that journal is devoted to descriptions of important medical ethics programs at major medical schools.

17. John K. Roth and Michael Berenbaum, eds., *The Holocaust: Religious and Philosophical Implications* (New York: Paragon House, 1989), p. xxiv.

15

Toward a Comprehensive Philosophy for Medicine

In this book we have examined one facet of the moral philosophy of medicine—the place virtue theory occupies—and its relationship to principle- and duty-based theories. This is far from a complete rendition of the practical structure requisite for an integral or complete moral philosophy peculiar to medicine. Such a moral philosophy would require that the principles, duties, and virtues appropriate to right and good medical morality themselves be grounded in something more fundamental—in a theory of medicine or some theory of the moral order (its ontology, epistemology, and axiology) as they relate and are applied to a theory of medicine.

Today we are a long way from such a comprehensive moral philosophy. There are many obstacles—both conceptual and practical—to its attainment. For one thing, there is no agreement about which of the great moral traditions should be the source for the principles that should guide the moral behavior of physicians. Nor is there consensus on what it means to have moral knowledge—that is, whether moral knowledge is an illusion or whether it has some basis outside out the subject who claims it. Moreover, since the object of the concerns of both medicine and morality is the human being, we might expect a moral philosophy of medicine to have its roots in some agreed-upon conception of the human being, of the ends of individual and collective human existence. Without a philosophical anthropology, the widespread talk about "human values," their definitions, or their order or priority must lack an axiological substratum.

Much of the ferment in medical ethics, the skepticism about and disarticulation of the Hippocratic tradition, are attributable to the wide divergence of opinion about these determinants of an integral medical ethic. As MacIntyre and others have shown, this divergence has a long history, but it was not made explicit until the mid-1960s in the United States. For a time, it seemed that the device of *prima facie* principles might suffice to paper over the gaps that had opened in general and medical-moral theory. However, in recent years, as the criticism of *prima facie* principles has grown in intensity, alternate theories have been propounded to make up for the perceived deficiencies of principles. But there is little likelihood that any one of these alternatives will be sufficient either to replace principles entirely or to provide the conceptual grounding a moral philosophy of medicine requires.

In this last chapter, we will examine the philosophical structure of traditional ethics, the impact *prima facie* principles have had on its content and methodology, the criticism now being leveled against *prima facie* principles by competing theories, and the way the unsettled state of philosophy itself as an enterprise further complicates any attempt to construct a comprehensive theory and practice of medical ethics in the foreseeable future.

The Origins: Revisiting the Hippocratic Ethic

The backbone of medical ethics for 2500 years was the Hippocratic ethic, which consists of the Oath and the deontological books of the Hippocratic corpus.[1] Philosophically, the ethics of the corpus is a mosaic of moral precepts written at different times and influenced by most of the major schools of ancient Greek philosophy. The Oath, which includes most of the genuinely moral precepts, is considered to be strongly but not exclusively influenced by Pythagorean philosophy.[2] It contains most of the genuinely ethical precepts like the obligations of beneficence, non-maleficence, and confidentiality; the prohibition of abortion, euthanasia, and sexual relationships with patients; and the exhortation to lead a "pure, holy" life. The deontological books, on the other hand, are more in the realm of etiquette, or what is expected of a prudent gentleman. They emphasize rules about dress, gossip, reputation, comportment, cleanliness, truth-telling, consultations with other physicians, and the physician's education. Later Stoic influences added an emphasis on duty[3] and compassion.[4]

The method of decision-making consisted of judgments about whether a given form of conduct was in conformity with these precepts. There is no evidence of critical analysis of moral choice in the modern sense. This is characteristic of Aristotelian, Socratic, and Platonic moral philosophy in general. These philosophers focused on the overall aims of the moral life like the good, justice, and cultivation of the virtues. In this view, the virtuous physician was one habitually disposed to act in conformity with the virtues of courage, temperance, and justice and with the moral precepts of the Oath. As we saw, the key virtue was *phronesis*, the virtue of practical judgment, whereby the physician was able to discern the right and good thing to do in a particular situation. This was reemphasized by us in our examination of the virtues in Part II of this book.

Greek medicine and philosophy cross-fertilized each other. Socrates, Plato, and Aristotle used medicine extensively as a pedagogic tool, particularly as a model of the ethical use of knowledge.[5] They found in it a source of analogies in which the health of the body (medicine) was likened to the health of the soul (philosophy). Likewise, medicine's norms of health became a model for the norms of the moral life. So close was the identification between medicine and philosophy that the Hippocratic physicians at one point had to assert their independence.[6]

What is interesting in all of this is that the ethic of the Hippocratic corpus never became a subject of formal philosophical scrutiny on its own. Neither Plato nor Aristotle, nor the Stoics after them, ever produced a treatise specifically devoted to the ethics of the physician. This was true even in the Hellenic period, when the major philosophical schools strongly influenced medicine's theories of disease and health.[7]

Philosophers ancient and modern, of course, have always written on such fundamental ethical issues as abortion, euthanasia, suicide, death, and infanticide. These problems would fit the rubric of biomedical ethics as it is used today. But the ethics of the physician–patient relationship, the fulcrum on which the decisions of the physician and the well-being of the patient are balanced, was not systematically justified or derived in any formal way.

Even physicians who were philosophers, Alcmaeon and Empedocles in the ancient world or John Locke and William James in the modern one, said little, as philosophers, about the ethics of the profession in which they were trained. Karl Jaspers did devote two informal essays to the physician–patient relationship but wrote no genuine moral inquiry into medical ethics.[8]

This is not the place to trace the historical modifications of the Hippocratic ethic as it came into contact with the great religious traditions.[9] With minor modifications to remove traces of its pagan origins, the Hippocratic ethic remained essentially unchanged in the writings of the most influential physicians like Percival[10] and Gregory[11] in England, and Hooker[12] in America. The basic Hippocratic texts, along with Stoic notions of duty and virtue, congruent elements in the Jewish and Christian Bibles and teachings, and the noblesse oblige expected of a gentleman all were intermingled. This is the synthesis that inspired the first Code of the American Medical Association in 1847. While it was progressively attenuated in successive versions of the code, it remained the moral background against which most American and British physicians made, and still make, their ethical choices.

The mosaic of philosophical constructs that make up the Hippocratic synthesis was, for almost its entire history, a taken-for-granted ethical system. It came to be examined critically only in the mid-1960s as part of the general upheaval of moral values that occurred in American society as the result of a series of societal changes—better education of the public; the spread of participatory democracy through the civil rights, feminist, and consumer movements; decline in the sense of communally shared values; a heightened sense of ethnicity; and a distrust of authority and institutions of all kinds. These forces were accentuated in medicine by the specialization, fragmentation, institutionalization, and depersonalization of health care that occurred simultaneously with an expansion in the number and complexity of medical ethical issues.

The net result was to cast doubt on the traditional moral moorings of society in general, and medicine in particular, and to create a demand for alternative models of teaching and practicing medical ethics. The way was paved for serious philosophical inquiry because the questions being raised were ultimately questions of moral value, and these were the perennial questions to which moral philosophers addressed themselves.

Three forms of resolution suggest themselves in the presence of this polarity: restoration, deconstruction, or reconstruction. Let us look at each in the light of the challenges posed by trying to wed a virtue-based ethic and a principled-ethic.

The restoration of medical ethics to its presumed pristine rectitude is favored by many, particularly older physicians. To them, the sum and substance of medical ethics is contained in the Hippocratic Oath, and its status is quasi-scriptural. Often the proponents of this view are concerned with restoring some proscription or other without looking critically at the remaining items in the Oath. One may favor, for example, the restoration of the proscription against abortion but may nonetheless agree that the Oath, and the whole Hippocratic corpus as well, is inadequate to deal with the range of ethical issues that confront us today. Some of its principles are simply not morally-defensible—like the benign authoritarianism, the refusal to disclose the patient's condition, the absence of social responsibility, and the absolute ban on violations of confidentiality. These items need to change not because the times have changed, but because they were morally insecure in the first place.

What then about deconstruction, the disassembly of the ancient edifice? Should we not see the ethics of medicine, and especially the medical relationship, as a "text" upon which, like any text lifted out of its context, we may impose truth and meaning as we read them? This is a growing tendency today, especially with respect to euthanasia, abortion, and sexual relationships with patients. In a deconstructionist view, the text means what we think it means or what we want it to mean. Doctor and patient, in this view, are free to deconstruct the traditional text and renegotiate one of their own. There is a text or ethic for each situation and each dyad of physician and patient. The result is a normless, constantly redefined, nihilistic reading of a text—which is to say that there really is no text at all. The only "moral code" that exists is the assurance that doctor and patient have the freedom to give their own private meanings to the text. If there is any text, it is only a backdrop against which individual parties to the relationship examine their own motives and actions—whenever the necessary link is deconstructed, artificially, between text and its context.

The routes of restoration and deconstruction are equally untenable. What is needed instead is a reconstruction of medical ethics, a reexamination of its foundations for what in the tradition is morally valid, what is invalid, what is missing, what ought to be changed, and what ought to be added. This is an endeavor still to be undertaken. It involves a critical assessment of ethical principles concerning the nature of the medical relationship, the kind of human activity it represents, the specific obligations that arise from that activity for both the physician and the patient, and the relation of the virtues of the agents to these features. In a way, this process moves medical ethics from the realm of moral assertion to that of reasoned ethical discourse. Where such a reasoned examination will lead will, of course, bring us back to some of the unresolved first-order questions to which we referred at the outset of our book, namely, how medicine functions as a moral community, how this life experience gives rise to virtues and moral character, how the ends of medicine shape both the training and practice of physicians and the virtues we expect of them, and how the virtues relate to moral rules and principles?

In any case, the questions we have raised cannot be answered without some model of medical ethics that has more structure than transitory norms or hermeneutic laxity would permit.

The Ascendance of Prima Facie Principles

With the erosion of the Hippocratic synthesis, some physicians sought guidance in court decisions or legislation, or took a nihilistic view of ethics entirely. Most, however, recognized the dangers of confusing law or economics with ethics and of reducing professional ethics to nothing more than personal opinion. For them, moral philosophy had certain attractive features. It offered a systematic and relatively objective way to approach ethical dilemmas. Its analytical rigor appealed to academic clinicians who were becoming aware of the need to address ethical dilemmas and to teach medical ethics in a new way. Its freedom from faith-ommitments suited the moral—and religious—heterogeneity of medical student bodies.

The philosophers who began to examine medical ethics brought a variety of well-established moral traditions to bear on their reflections, most usually some variant of act- or rule-based deontology or consequentialism. But one theory, W.D. Ross' theory of *prima facie* principles, had a particular appeal to physicians and soon became the dominant way of "doing ethics."[13] This approach was adapted to medical ethics in the text that has most influenced clinicians, Beauchamp and Childress' *Principles of Biomedical Ethics.*[14]

Beauchamp and Childress recognized the difficulties of attaining agreement on the most fundamental foundations of ethics: the nature of the good, the ultimate sources of morality, and the epistemological status of moral knowledge. To bypass these problems, they followed the direction taken by W. D. Ross and opted for *prima facie* principles, that is, principles that should always be respected unless some strong countervailing reason exists that would justify overruling them. Four principles in this *prima facie* category were especially appropriate for medical ethics—nonmaleficence, beneficence, autonomy, and justice.

This tetrad of principles had the advantage of compatibility with deontological and consequentialist theories, and even with some aspects of virtue theory. It was applied quickly to the resolution of ethical dilemmas by medical ethicists, and especially by health professionals. For clinicians, this four-principle schema we examined in earlier chapters had several appeals. First, it promised to reduce some of the looseness and subjectivity that had characterized so many ethical debates; second, it provided fairly specific action guidelines; third, it offered an orderly way to "workup" an ethical problem in a way analogous to the clinical workup of a diagnostic or therapeutic problem; finally, it avoided direct confrontation with the intractably divisive issues of abortion, euthanasia, and the use of reproductive technologies.

In addition, two of the *prima facie* principles, beneficence and nonmaleficence, were identical to the Hippocratic obligations to act in the best interests of the patient and to avoid doing harm. On the other hand, two others—autonomy and justice—were unfamiliar and even, in some sense, antithetical to beneficence and nonmaleficence.

Autonomy directly contradicted the traditional authoritarianism and paternalism of the Hippocratic ethic, which gave no place to patient participation in clinical decisions. Modern physicians have had the greatest problems with this principle, since it often is interpreted erroneously as being in opposition to beneficence.[15] Physicians belatedly have come to accept the principle of autonomy largely because it is central to informed consent and consistent with the individualistic temper, with its emphasis on privacy and self-governance, that had set the initial metamorphosis of medical ethics in motion. Many clinicians, however, still are not fully convinced of the soundness of autonomy as a primary principle. Many fear its absolutization, which may override good medical judgment or encourage detachment on the part of the physician.

Of the four principles, justice is the most remote from traditional medical ethics. Despite its prominence in the philosophies of Plato and Aristotle, justice received no specific attention in the Hippocratic ethic, which focused on the welfare of individual patients and not of society. Historically, justice entered medical ethics much later, usually in relation to the physician's forensic duties.

In recent years, justice has entered medical ethics more forcibly as disparities in the distribution of health care have become more apparent. The possibility that physicians may become agents primarily of fiscal or social purpose rather than of the patient increases daily. Acting as a gatekeeper or rationer poses a worrisome conflict of obligations for many traditionally minded clinicians. Nonetheless, Rawls' sophisticated contractarian theory of justice and his lexical ordering of obligations and principles relative to distributive justice have placed justice squarely in the forefront of medical ethics.[16] Our judgment is that justice as an intrinsic virtue of medicine still requires more analysis than we could give it in this book—despite our admiration for the work of Daniels, Veatch, and MacIntyre in this respect.[17]

The four-principle approach has been taught to thousands of health professionals through the most popular intensive bioethics course, conducted annually by the faculty of the Kennedy Institute of Ethics for the last seventeen years. Through its 200 or so graduates per year, this course has had a strong influence on the teaching and research of health professionals and ethicists who teach in medical schools, colleges and universities, or consult in clinical settings. Many younger health professionals have learned ethics from those graduates, who now head up many of the centers of bioethics. The four-principle tradition is now so widely accepted that some of its more whimsical critics have labeled it a "mantra," applied automatically and without sound moral grounding.[18]

The authors of the four-principle approach were, of course, well aware of the limitations of Ross' system of *prima facie* obligations—for example, the difficulties of putting any set of abstract principles into practice in particular cases, or the difficulty of reducing conflicts between *prima facie* principles or within a single principle without some hierarchical or lexical ordering of the principles. Ross' rather vague formula of taking the action that gives the best balance of right over wrong begs those questions. We still need some principle by which to measure the appropriateness of the balance.

To accommodate those shortcomings, Beauchamp and Childress proposed four requirements that must be met to justify "infringements" of a *prima facie* principle or obligation: (1) the moral objective sought is realistic; (2) no morally preferable alternative is available; (3) the least infringement possible must be sought; and (4) the agent must act to minimize the effects of infringement.[19] These authors hope in this way to steer a course between the absolutism of principles and the relativism of situation ethics. Their guidelines are helpful but do not eradicate the inherent limitations of any set of *prima facie* principles that is not lexically ordered.

The Growing Criticism of Principlism and of the Virtue Theory Alternative

These limitations of principlism were the subject of serious criticism in an issue of the *Journal of Medicine and Philosophy*.[20] In that issue, Brody calls the four principles "mid-level" principles, meaning that they are themselves in need of rational justification and of a firmer grounding in one of the great moral traditions.[21] Clouser and Gert decry the lack of a unifying moral theory that would tie the principles together and give them the conceptual grounding they need.[22] Were such a theory available, it would make the principles unnecessary. Holmes, like MacIntyre earlier, contends that philosophical ethics itself is of limited value.[23] He calls for "moral wisdom" for which philosophy does not prepare us. Gustafson argues that philosophy is an insufficient tool for confronting the broad agenda of biomedical ethics. He calls for the inclusion of prophetic, narrative, and public policy elements in the discourse. These, he feels, are more suited than principles to resolution of key ethical issues in health care.[24]

Other criticisms of the four principles come largely from outside the philosophical community. Principles, it is said, are too abstract, too rationalistic, and too removed from the moral and psychological milieu in which moral choices are actually made; principles ignore a person's character, life story, cultural background, and gender. They imply a technical perfection in moral decisions which is frustrated by the psychological uniqueness of each moral agent or act.

Many remedies are offered to replace, prioritize, complement, or supplement *prima facie* principles. Englehardt, for example, places autonomy in the first order of priority[25] ahead of beneficence:[26] We favor beneficence in trust for that position;[27] others choose non-maleficence or justice. Additional alternatives to principle-based theories include an ethic based in virtue, caring, "experience," casuistry, or a return to theological and biblical sources as the only reliable grounding for medical morals.

The growing support for alternatives to principle-based medical ethics indicates clearly that the metamorphosis that has already been so rapid and profound is far from complete. How these theories will influence the future of medical ethics is problematic. But it is clear that in the next decade, physicians who have just accommodated their thinking to the four-principle approach must now sort out the place of each of the proposed alternatives. They must decide whether principlism can or should survive, and in what form, and to what degree alternative theories should complement or supplant it.

Prospective on a Metamorphosis

Will Principles Survive?

It is clear that principlism in its present form is unlikely to survive unscathed through the next decade. But its limitations notwithstanding, we do not believe principles will disappear for several reasons.

First, principles—that is to say, fundamental sources from which specific action-guides like duties or rules derive and are justified—are implicit in any ethical system. The Hippocratic ethic, for example, was virtue-based, but its action-guides were rules and principles. Second, there are equally serious limitations to any alternative theory to principlism. Third, the necessity and utility of principles becomes increasingly evident when we try to apply the alternative theories to actual cases: Finally, principles inherently are not incompatible with other theories. The real question, as old as moral philosophy itself, is how to go from universal principles to individual moral decisions and back again.

Surely the character of the agent is crucial to medical ethics, since the health professional is the agent who interprets and applies whatever theory is used. Virtue was the implicit and dominant theory in traditional medical ethics until the beginning of the thirty-year period we have been considering. It would, however, be simplistic to urge a complete return to virtue as the basis for medical ethics. MacIntyre has shown brilliantly how irretrievable is the metaphysical consensus that virtue theories require.[28] Virtue ethics by itself does not provide sufficiently clear action-guides; it is too private, too prone to individual definitions of virtue or the virtuous person.

Virtue theory must be anchored in some prior theory of the right and the good and of human nature in terms of which the virtues can be defined. It also requires a community of values to sustain its practice. In an integrated medical ethics, virtue and character will be folded into any future version of biomedical ethics. This will require a conceptual link with duties, rules, consequences, and moral psychology, in which the virtue of prudence plays a special role.[29]

Besides virtue theory explored in this book, a second alternative attractive to health professionals is the ethic of caring, certainly a prime aim of healing relationships.[30] Adherents of this view hold that women are more caring than men in the way they approach ethical decisions. They are presumed to be more interested in relationships than individual assertions, in reconciliation rather than in winning arguments, in attachment rather than detachment, in nurturing rather than dominating, and so on.

Few would or could deny the necessity of an account of caring in any comprehensive theory of medical ethics. But there are empirical and philosophical objections to this model of moral reasoning.[31] Gender differences, for example, may be based more in social class, culture, self-image, and personal ideals than in the developmental psychology of Freud or Kohlberg.[32] These gender differences and their contribution to medical ethics surely should be factored into any future biomedical ethic. But "caring" is subject to such a wide variety of interpretations that it too needs some grounding in a principle or rule to be a trustworthy guide to specific ethical decision-making. Moral psychology is an adjutant to but not a replacement for ethical principles.

A third alternative, particularly appealing to clinicians because it focuses on concrete and particular cases, is the revival of casuistry.[33] The casuist looks for cases that are obvious examples of a principle, that is, a case on which there is sure to be a high degree of agreement among most, if not all, observers. The casuist then moves from the clear to more dubious cases and puts them in order by paradigm and analogy under some principle. Casuistry, therefore, does not eschew principles, nor is it incompatible with them. Its nemesis is the *absolutization* of principles.

Casuists try to circumvent the moral pluralism of contemporary society. But casuistry is a product of the cultures of the Roman and Middle Ages, when there was consensus on certain principles (the Decalogue, for example). It runs into difficulties when there is no such consensus, since the moral viewpoint of a society defines what it considers a dilemma or a paradigm case. Casuistry, as it was used in Catholic moral theology, functioned within the context of a common belief in God, the destiny of humankind, the acceptance of the principles of double effect, of totality, and the theory of probabilism.[34] No such consensus exists, even among Roman Catholics, in today's morally heterogeneous society. Casuistry can function as a method of case analysis, but not as a reliable guide to moral theory or practice.

Clearly, the proposed alternatives to principlism can enrich any theory of medical ethics. None is independent of principles, rules, or obligations, without which they succumb to the debilities of subjectivism and relativism. What is required is some comprehensive philosophical underpinning for medical ethics that will link the great moral traditions with principles and rules and with the new emphasis on moral psychology. This obviously calls for more than an affable eclecticism.

The elaboration of a new underpinning for medical ethics will be greatly complicated by the parlous state of contemporary philosophy and ethics and the strong current of nihilism and skepticism in both fields. In philosophy, for example, Rorty denies the possibility of arriving at any truths through philosophy and the relevance of any theory of reality.[35] Derrida likewise denies that there is any truth, only the appearances, and words to which we impute whatever meaning they may have.[36] Williams takes the same skeptical view of ethics and moral accountability.[37] These writers demolish philosophy, theology, and ethics simultaneously in full capitulation to the Nietzschean legacy.[38] For Nietzsche, the idea of one truth was an illusion: all we are capable of discussing are multiple truths seen from many perspectives that are incommensurable with each other.[39]

Such radical relativism is reinforced by the worldwide surge of cultural hegemony in morality. In this view, the medical ethic that has supplanted the Hippocratic ethic is a Western product and is incompatible on various ground with other cultures, particularly with reference to autonomy. As the Western version comes into contact with other cultures, we can expect sharper definitions of points of conflict and agreement.[40]

There is in medical ethics more hope for a better grounding of principles, rules, virtues, and moral psychology than in any other field of ethics. That hope rests on the universality of the experiences of illness and healing, and on the proximate and ultimate aims of medicine. The advantages of the four-principle approach can be preserved and even given lexical ordering, as we argued in our early chapters, if they are grounded in the realities of the physician–patient relationship.

Models of Medical Ethics

Whatever our positions may be on the fundamental propadeutic questions and moral presuppositions, we have examined the debate about virtue-based and principle-based ethics on the basis of the physician–patient relationship and its fundamental purposes. There are many models of medical ethics now under consideration, but we summarize our argument for an integrated medical ethics with two generic types—those that emphasize patient autonomy and those that emphasize beneficence as the organizing ethical principle.

Autonomy-Based Models

The most popular models among ethicists and jurists today are those that emphasize patient autonomy. They have arisen largely to counter the paternalism of the traditional Hippocratic model. They have served well in exposing the moral deficiencies of benign authoritarianism, especially as it pertains to decisions about death and dying. They combat the fears of overzealous treatment and of loss of control of one's life when death seems imminent or inevitable.

Autonomy models come in two general forms—a consumer model and a negotiated contract model. In the consumer model, the physician provides the facts about the alternatives, and the patient assesses each alternative in terms of his own values. The doctor is only a technical assistant. Her values and her judgments of the patient's values are not relevant. Patient autonomy is the central and overriding principle. The patient's intention is determinative in intending death, and so are the intentions of his valid surrogate.

In the contractual or negotiated model, physician and patient discuss their mutual values, those related to health, and those related to their moral systems. The physician acts to varying degrees as an informant, interpreter, or teacher, eliciting and balancing the patient's wishes. Physicians and patients are autonomous in that they agree to pursue a course together and freely enter into a contractual relationship with each other. They may share the intention to hasten death by euthanasia or assisted suicide, and this intention is negotiable between them but is of no concern to third parties, since patient and physician are always free to contract with each other as they choose.

Autonomy models are largely instrumental, transactional, and procedural. They need not conform to any external set of norms. The contracting parties create their own 'text' and give it the ethical meaning they choose. They bypass the fundamental moral questions and context entirely and render the idea of right and wrong intentions irrelevant. They are *ipso facto* deconstructionists.

To accept an autonomy model is to accept the demise of any notion of a common morality of medicine, except insofar as that morality is defined by the law of contracts. Principles—like autonomy itself or beneficence—would be *prima facie* principles only to the extent and in the terms defined by the contracting parties.

The dangers of autonomy models are serious. They tend to moral atomism and moral anarchy. They are actually self-defeating, since the contracting parties are not equals either in knowledge or in power. They end up extinguishing autonomy in the name of autonomy, since in subtle ways, for example in euthanasia, the physician's values and interpretations of what is intolerable suffering, what is worthwhile life, and what is the right thing to do will inevitably insinuate themselves into the terms and performance of the contract. Without some moral construct specific to the experience of illness and built upon the primacy of the patient's welfare, the doctor's will and intent will, in the majority of the cases, prevail.

A sounder model morally, one that would protect the autonomy of both physician and patient but would place both under the constraint of beneficence, is preferable and more responsive to the realities of the clinical situation.

An End-Oriented Beneficence Model

The physician–patient relationship centers on a unique human experience: the experience of illness, something that no two persons experience identically. This relationship begins when a sick person seeks the expert knowledge and skill of a physician who can help her to attain specific ends that she deems worthwhile. These ends are three. In the long term, the end is health; in the shorter term, the end is cure, containment, amelioration, or prevention of illness, pain, and disability. The most proximate and immediate end of this relationship is a technically correct and morally good healing decision for and with a particular patient. These three ends give the medical relationship its special architectonic, such that the moral quality of the physician's (and the patient's) actions is definable in terms of the extent to which those actions facilitate or obstruct the realization of the ends of medicine.

In this sense, then, the ethic of medicine we promulgate is a teleological ethic. This is not a consequentialist ethic in the modern sense but a teleological one in the classical sense—an ethic whose content is determined by the specific ends of medical activity. These goals and purposes are embedded in the very activity that gives medicine its distinctive character and distinguishes it from other kinds of human activity. These ends, in turn, define the moral character and composite of virtues we have detailed in this book. It is in this orientation towards specific ends— the three ends of medicine, for example, health, cure, and care of a specific illness, and a right and good healing decision—that the intentions and virtues of the doctor and patient become morally pertinent.

This architectonic constitutes a framework within which moral intent, moral choice, and moral action are to be judged. These are the human, existential, and personal phenomena that give a special moral climate to medical ethics.

The internal morality of medicine consists, then, of the principles, duties, obligations, and moral character that arise from a consideration of the special nature of the medical relationship expressed in two triads—the three ends of medicine and the three phenomena of the medical relationship. These triads provide the conceptual basis for the duties that devolve on both physician and patient in their joint pursuit of the ends specific to medicine.

Thus, the principle of beneficence and nonmaleficence states that the physician must so act that the best interests—that is to say, the good—of the patient are the primary goal. Effacement of self-interest to a certain degree and enhancing the good of the patient are obligations defined by this principle. Any intentional harm inflicted upon the person of the patient is a maleficent act that, by definition, defeats the ends of medicine, which are healing and helping.

The principle of autonomy requires that the values, wishes, and preferences of the patient be determinative in medical choice. This principle imposes the obligation to invite, enhance, and protect the patient's decision-making capacity. Indeed, to violate the patient's autonomy is in itself a maleficent act, since it is a direct assault on the patient's humanity, which is linked to full operation of his reason and judgment. Informed consent is an obvious *sine qua non* of respect for patient autonomy.

Justice is a third principle in the internal morality of medicine because it requires the physician to act in such a way that she renders to the patient what is owed— namely, proper fulfillment of the ends of medicine and responsive to the peculiar existential state that binds physician and patient in the medical relationship. Justice also requires a proper balancing of the claims of the patient, especially his autonomy claims against those of third parties and those of the physician herself.

In a similar fashion, the subsidiary principles of truth telling, promise keeping, and confidentiality can be derived from the ends of medicine and the phenomena special to **the healing relationship**. If our primary line of argument is coherent, the subsidiary principles should follow as well.

The internal morality of medicine also defines the principles and duties that should bind the patient. It often is forgotten that the medical relationship, like any moral relationship, is one of mutual obligation. Thus, the patient enters the relationship to attain the three ends of medicine we have described—health, cure, and care—as well as an immediate decision that is technically correct and good.[41]

The patient shares with the physician, therefore, an obligation to act according to principles and in fulfillment of duties that will attain and not obstruct these ends. To enter into a medical relationship obligates the patient in several ways: the patient must provide honestly the data the physician needs, comply with the agreed-upon regimen, disclose conflicting advice or doubts about the advice given, consider the needs of the physician as a human being, and respect the physician's autonomy and moral values.

In a similar manner, the virtues of the good physician and patient can be related to the special circumstances of the medical relationship. In this view, the physician's virtues are habitual dispositions to act in such a way that the ends of medicine are enhanced and enriched. Honesty, justice, benevolence, humility, and courage are virtues of the good physician, as they are of the good patient, since these virtues dispose both parties to act well in relation to the ends of medicine.

Conclusion

If current debates in medical ethics are to shape the character and virtues of the physician of the next century, then a compressed moral analysis in terms of rules, principles, and public policy must be expanded by attention to the goals of medicine, the ends of the clinical encounter, and the virtues we may expect of individual physicians and patients in the coming decades.

However parlous the state of contemporary postmodern philosophy may be, plain people, like doctors and patients, will ask, "What is the right and good thing for me to do? What is *the* good for patients, and what kinds of actions will achieve it?"[42] No one making practical ethical decisions can escape these questions, even those philosophers who are professional skeptics or nihilists. There are "no atheists in foxholes," and there are no patients who are truly nihilists or total skeptics when their own health or welfare is at stake.

In the last thirty years, the philosophical underpinnings of medical ethics have undergone a profound metamorphosis. Just where that metamorphosis will lead in the next decade, when philosophy and ethics themselves are being eroded, is problematic. Physicians and other health workers must be familiar with shifts in contemporary moral philosophy if they are to help restructure the ethics of their profession. They all need to provide a "reality check" on the nihilism and skepticism of contemporary philosophy. Medical ethics is too ancient and too essential a reality for physicians, patients, and society to be left entirely to the fortuitous currents of philosophical fashion.

Our examination of the issues arising from a virtue ethic in medicine is only the first step in this enormous challenge.

Notes

1. Hippocrates, *Hippocrates (I and II)*, trans. by W. H. L. Jones, Loeb Classical Library (No. 147 and 148) (Cambridge, MA: Harvard University Press, 1972 and 1981: *The Oath* (I, 289–302); *Precepts* (I, 303–333); *Law* (II, 263–265); *Decorum* (II, 279–299); and *The Physician* (II, 311–313).

2. P. Carrick, *Medical Ethics in Antiquity* (Dordrecht: D. Reidel, 1985), p. 163.

3. Cicero, "De Officiis," *Cicero* (XXI), trans. Walter Miller, Loeb Classical Library (No. 30) (Cambridge, MA: Harvard University Press, 1975).

4. Edmund D. Pellegrino and Alice A. Pellegrino, "Humanism and Ethics in Roman Medicine: Translation and Commentary on a Text of Scribonius Largus," *Literature and Medicine* 7 (1988):22–38.

5. W. Jaeger, *Paidea: The Ideals of Greek Culture,* Vol. 3 (New York: Oxford University Press, 1945), pp. 3–45.

6. Hippocrates, "The Art," *Hippocrates (II)*, trans. W. H. L. Jones, Loeb Classical Library (No. 148) (Cambridge, MA: Harvard University Press, 1981), pp. 185–217.

7. R. O. Moon, *Hippocrates and His Successors in Relation to the Philosophy of Their Time* (New York: Longmans, Green, 1923), pp. 91–162.

8. K. Jaspers, *Philosophy and the World: Selected Essays and Lectures* (Chicago: Regnery Gateway, 1963), pp. 153–167.

9. O. Temkin, *Hippocrates in a World of Pagans and Christians* (Baltimore, MD: Johns Hopkins University Press, 1991).

10. Thomas Percival, *Medical Ethics* (London: S. Russell, 1803).

11. J. Gregory, *Lectures on the Duties and Qualifications of a Physician* (London: Strahan and T. Cadell, 1772).

12. W. Hooker, *Physician and the Patient or, a Practical View of the Mutual Duties, Relations, and Interests of the Medical Profession and the Community* (New York: Arno Press and the New York Times, 1972).

13. W. D. Ross, *The Right and the Good* (Indianapolis: Hackett, 1988), p. 19.

14. Tom L. Beauchamp and James F. Childress, *Principles of Biomedical Ethics,* 3d ed. (New York: Oxford University Press, 1989).

15. Tom L. Beauchamp and Laurence B. McCullough, *Medical Ethics, the Moral Responsibilities of Physicians* (Englewood Cliffs, NJ: Prentice-Hall, 1984), pp. 22–51; Hippocrates, "The Oath," in *Hippocrates (I),* trans. W. H. S. Jones Loeb Classical Library (No. 147) (Cambridge, MA: Harvard University Press, 1972), pp. 299–302.

16. John Rawls, *A Theory of Justice* (Cambridge, MA: Harvard University Press, 1971), pp. 302–303.

17. Norman Daniels, *Just Health Care* (New York/Cambridge: Cambridge University Press, 1985); Robert Veatch, *A Theory of Medical Ethics* (New York: Basic Books, 1981); Alasdair MacIntyre, *Whose Justice? Which Rationality?* (Notre Dame, IN: University of Notre Dame Press, 1988).

18. K. Danner Clouser and Bernard Gert, "A Critique of Principlism," *Journal of Medicine and Philosophy* 15(2) (April 1990):219–236.

19. Beauchamp and Childress, *Principles of Biomedical Ethics,* p. 53.

20. See the issue of *Journal of Medicine and Philosophy* 15(2) (April 1990).

21. Baruch A. Brody, "Quality of Scholarship in Bioethics," *Journal of Medicine and Philosophy* 15(2) (April 1990):161–178.

22. Clouser and Gert, "Critique of Principlism."

23. R. L. Holmes, "The Limited Relevance of Analytical Ethics to the Problems of Bioethics," *Journal of Medicine and Philosophy* 15(2) (April 1990):143–160; Alasdair MacIntyre, "A Crisis in Moral Philosophy: Why Is the Search for Foundations So Frustrating?", *Knowing and Valuing,* ed. H. T. Engelhardt and D. Callahan (Hastings-on-Hudson, NY: Hastings Center, 1980), pp. 18–43.

24. J. M. Gustafson, "Moral Discourse About Medicine: A Variety of Forms," *Journal of Medicine and Philosophy* 15(2) (April 1990):125–142.

25. H. T. Engelhardt, *The Foundations of Bioethics* (New York: Oxford University Press, 1986).

26. H.T. Engelhardt and M. A. Rie, "Morality for the Medical-Industrial Complex— A Code of Ethics for the Mass Marketing of Health Care," *New England Journal of Medicine* 319(16) (October 1988):1086–1089.

27. E. D. Pellegrino and D. C. Thomasma, *For the Patient's Good: The Restoration of Beneficence in Health Care* (New York: Oxford University Press, 1988).

28. A. MacIntyre, *After Virtue,* 2d ed. (Notre Dame, IN: University of Notre Dame Press, 1988).

29. A. MacIntyre, *Three Rival Versions of Moral Enquiry* (Notre Dame, IN: University of Notre Dame Press, 1990), p. 139.

30. H. Nelson, "Against Caring," *Journal of Clinical Ethics* 3(1) (Spring, 1992):8–

15; C. Gilligan *In a Different Voice: Psychological Theory and Women's Development* (Cambridge, MA: Harvard University Press, 1983).

31. N. Noddings, *Caring, A Feminine Approach to Ethics and Moral Education* (Berkeley: University of California Press, 1984); S. Callahan, *In Good Conscience: Reason and Emotion in Moral Decision-Making* (San Francisco: Harper-Collins, 1991).

32. O. Flanagan, *Varieties of Moral Personality: Ethics and Psychological Realism* (Cambridge, MA: Harvard University Press, 1991).

33. A.R. Jonsen and S. Toulmin, *The Abuse of Casuistry: A History of Moral Reasoning* (Berkeley: University of California Press, 1988).

34. K.M. Wildes, "The Priesthood of Bioethics and the Return of Casuistry," *Journal of Medicine and Philosophy* 18(1) (in press).

35. R. Rorty, *Philosophy and the Mirror of Nature* (Princeton, NJ: Princeton University Press, 1979).

36. G. B. Madison, "Coping with Nietzsche's Legacy—Rorty, Derrida, Gadamer," *Philosophy Today* 34(1) (Spring 1992):3–19.

37. B. Williams, *Ethics and the Limits of Philosophy* (Cambridge, MA: Harvard University Press, 1985); B. Williams, *Moral Luck* (Cambridge, MA: Harvard University Press, 1981).

38. Madison, "Coping."

39. MacIntyre, *Three Rival Versions*.

40. H. E. Flack and E. D. Pellegrino, eds., *African-American Perspectives in Biomedical Ethics* (Washington, DC: Georgetown University Press, 1992); E. D. Pellegrino, P. Mazzarella, and P. Corsi, eds., *Transcultural Dimensions in Medical Ethics* (Frederick, MD.: University Publishing Group, in press).

41. Pellegrino and Thomasma, *For the Patient's Good*, pp. 99–110.

42. A. MacIntyre, "Plain Persons and Moral Philosophy: Rules, Virtues, and Goods," *American Catholic Philosophical Quarterly* 46(1) (Winter, 1992):1–19.

Index